EASY LIVING LOW-CARB COOKING

How many low-carb cookbooks have you looked at (or bought) where you've said, "You know, there's a lot of good recipes here, but who has time to make any of these?" Some low-carb cookbooks have recipes that are too exotic or just not practical to make at the end of a long day. Well as a low-carber who loves to cook, I felt the same way. Until I found the first edition of Easy Living Low-Carb Cooking, four years ago, I thought most low-carb cookbooks were impractical. From the day we first started selling the cookbook, it was always a best seller. When Tracy and Theresa told me they weren't going to reprint the cookbook anymore, I snatched it up and I'm very happy to present it to you.

These are recipes I can and want to make! Whether you're a working mom or a low-carb bachelor (like me!) these are great tasting recipes that are easy to make. Country Fried Steak, Chinese Cole Slaw, Peanut Butter Pie - doesn't sound like dieting does it!

I was also happy to get to know Tracy and Theresa. These are real working moms who know what their families want to eat - real American dishes that just happen to be low-carb. Each one of these recipes have been made for their families and have their seal of approval!

I hope you enjoy the recipes in this book. In fact, I hope you are able to use these recipes as the basis of your own meals or make some variations on them - that's the fun of cooking - being able to start with a great recipe and make it your own. If you have any questions about this cookbook, please email me at: **andrew@carbsmart.com**.

Sincerely,
Andrew S. DiMino
President and Founder
CarbSmart, Inc.
www.carbsmart.com

Copyright 1998, 2002 CarbSmart, Inc.

All rights reserved. No part of this book may be reproduced or transmitted in any form or by any means, electronic or mechanical, including photocopying, recording, or by any other information storage and retrieval system, without the express written permission of the Publisher, except where permitted by law.

CarbSmart, Inc.
1335 Greg Street, Suite 106
Sparks, NV 89431
775.356.1144 (phone)
775.356.1145 (fax)
www.carbsmart.com
publishing@carbsmart.com

Second Edition, Third Printing
Library of Congress Control Number: (currently being applied for)
ISBN: 0-9704931-0-X

Contents

Dedication 2

Introduction 3

Helpful Hints for Stocking Your Pantry and Freezer 7

Sample Menus 21

Appetizers and Snacks 25

Beverages 39

Salads and Dressings 43

Meaty Main Dishes 65
    Poultry 65
    Beef 85
    Pork 102
    Fish and Shellfish 113

Eggs and Cheese 119

Vegetables 129

Sauces 143

Desserts 151

Index 161

Dedication

We would like to dedicate this book first to the One who inspired, directed, and encouraged us throughout this project, the One to whom we dedicate our lives.

We would also like to dedicate this book to our husbands, children, family, and friends who provided so much help, support, and encouragement during the creation of this book. You have our lifelong love and endless thanks.

—Theresa and Tracy

Introduction

What an exciting culinary adventure low-carbohydrate eating and cooking has been! To think that we can feel better and lose weight while eating meat, cheese, eggs, and cream! When we discovered this philosophy of eating and cooking, we both did the proverbial "happy dance". We knew that our low-fat, high carbohydrate frustrations and disappointments were over.

This book was born out of a desire to expand our own eating avenues and to help those individuals who had been telling us, "Yes, this diet is great for losing weight, but.....what exactly can you eat?" or "If I have to eat another egg or piece of turkey breast I will just die." When we began questioning these individuals, "Have you tried this....or that? You know, you can eat this, this, this, and this...", they would look at us with shocked expressions and would relate to us their perception that low-carbohydrate eating was either incredibly bland or extremely gourmet, with little to no middle ground. We hope that this cookbook will dispell both notions and provide you with practical, affordable, convenient recipes and menu suggestions that both you and your family can live with.

Let us rush to say that this book is _not_ a diet program, but a companion text to any low-carbohydrate program that is on the market today. Whatever program you are following, we hope that you will find recipes here that will be compatible with your eating plan. We are not dieticians, nutritionists, trained chefs, or medical personnel of any kind. We are, however, busy working mothers who have families who are not necessarily following a low-carbohydrate diet, and all of us have to be fed out of a fairly modest food budget. Therefore, they eat what we eat. And we try really hard to make sure that they are happy with what we are eating.

The focus of this book is the weight loss phase of your eating plan. We attempted to include only those recipes whose carbohydrate count per serving was 0-6 grams. We used all information available to us to provide you with as accurate a count as possible. When in doubt, we rounded up so that the carbs might be a tad bit higher than reality. But, we figured "better safe than sorry".

We also tried to include as many convenience foods as we could that might save you some time and yet not throw you off the low-carbohydrate path. For some, this may be a bit surprising and perhaps disappointing, although we hope not. You see, we are real people trying to find our way through a high-carbohydrate world—which is not easy. We try to be as strict and as vigilant as we can without being "carbophobic". We may suggest a product or recipe from time to time that has some sugars or natural sweeteners in it, and yet at other times warn you about other products that have sugars in it. We hope to not be contradictory. Our reasoning for doing so is that the amount of sugar (or sweetener) in a particular product appeared to be minimal and did not raise the carb. count to an unrealistic level, and it is probably not a product that you will sit down and consume large amounts of at one time. However, other products may have a minimal amount and be something that you could conceivably eat or drink a large amount of at a time, and unwittingly sabotage yourself. If you know for yourself that you cannot tolerate even a small amount of sugar, etc. due to a hyper-sensitivity then you may choose to omit that product, ingredient, or recipe from your eating plan at this time. We are all different and what may be a "trigger" food for one person, may not affect another person at all. Our overall philosophy is this: Know what you're eating and try to minimize the use of carbohydrates (especially the simple carbs) in your diet, without living in a glass box. We are hopeful that others also have this same philosophy, and that you will go on this "tasteful adventure" with us.

Finally, you will find sprinkled throughout the book helpful hints, tips, thoughts, and comments that have been born out of our own experiences with this style of eating. If you have questions, comments, or concerns about where we got our information or how we arrived at a conclusion, please give us a call or write, and we will gladly share with you our sources.

Abbreviations that you will see throughout the remainder of the book
(For the more experienced cook, these may be very obvious, but we wanted to make clarification so that anyone—even the beginner cook—can understand and use our recipes)
carb/carbs—carbohydrates
g.—gram
T.—tablespoon
tsp.—teaspoon
C.—cup
lb.—pound
oz.—ounce
pkt.—packet
pkg.—package

Some Standard Measurement Conversions that we find useful:
3 tsp.=1 T.
16 T.=1 cup
2 C.=1 pint

Hints for Stocking Up

In order to make this (or any other) eating lifestyle consistent, we've found that we *had* to make it very convenient as well. If we didn't, and at the end of a hard day's work we found ourselves staring at the cabinets or refrigerator wondering, "O.K., what can we have tonight?" all too often the fast-food drive-throughs or the pizza deliveries would beckon to us.

In the next few pages, we would like to share with you some of the helpful tips and habits that we have incorporated into our shopping/stocking up routine to help make getting a meal on the table as quick and convenient as possible. If you have other ideas that we have, as yet, not thought of, please drop us a line—there is no such thing as being too organized or efficient, and we are always on the look-out for ways to make life easier.

The Pantry

The emphasis of low-carbohydrate eating plans leans (obviously) toward the meats and cheeses end of the spectrum, but you will find that you will develop a certain inventory of canned, bottled, and dry items that should always be kept on hand in your pantry to help you get a quick and tasty dinner on the table, especially when you don't feel like cooking. With a fairly set inventory in mind, if you happen to be a sale shopper, then you can really stock up when the prices are good, and be even further ahead of the game. As you find particular meals and menus becoming family favorites, you may want to consider having a written "check list" of grocery items posted to the inside of your cabinet door to make sure that you aren't running low of some essential ingredients. If you keep the following ingredients on hand, you will be able to create any recipe found in this book (just be sure you have *enough* of each ingredient before you begin):

Beverage Mixes
Coffee beans, Flavored (.8g/serving)
Herbal Teas, Celestial Seasonings (0g/serving)
Sugar-Free Beverage and Tea Mixes—Country-Time, Crystal
 Light, Lipton, (0-1g/serving)

Canned Meats
Armour Star Sliced Dried Beef (.4g/1oz serving)
Chunk Chicken (0g/1/4 C.—Hormel brand)
Corned Beef (0g/1/4 C. serving)
Crabmeat (0g/1/3 C.—S & W brand)
Deviled Ham (0g/1/4 C.—Underwood brand)
Tuna (0g. carbs/1/4 C. serving)

Canned Vegetables—We prefer fresh or frozen vegetables, but when time and convenience are of the essence, canned vegetables are very handy. Try to keep on hand:
Artichoke hearts (5g/3 pieces)
Bamboo Shoots (2.1g/1/2 C.)
Bean Sprouts (3g/2/3 C. serving)
Chop Suey vegetables (3g/2/3 C. serving)
Fancy Mixed Chinese Vegetables by La Choy (1g/2/3 C.serving)
Green beans, cut or French-style (5g. carbs/1/2 C. serving)
Green chiles—chopped and diced (1g /1oz. serving)
Mushrooms—sliced or stems and pieces (4g /1/4 C. serving)
Pimientos (3g/2oz. jar)
Sauerkraut (5g/1/2 C. serving)

Tomato Sauce (4g/1/4 C. serving)
(Canned Fruit—Crushed Pineapple Dole brand [17g/1/2 C.])

"Relish Tray Items"
Canned ripe, pitted olives (1g/5 olives)
Dill Pickles—whole and spears (1g/1oz serving)
Dill Pickle Relish (label states 0g/1T. serving)
Peppers, Banana or Pepperoncini (1g/1oz)
Pimiento-stuffed green olives (1g/5 olives)

Nuts and Nut Butters
Almonds, slivered or sliced (Paradise or White Swan brands—
    3g/1/4 C. serving; Planter's Gold Measure brand—
    11g/1/2 C. serving)
Macadamias (3.9g/1.0oz)
Pecan chips (Nut topping)—(9g/2oz pkg., approx. 1/2 C.)
Pecan halves—(9g/2oz pkg)
Pistachios, dry-roasted in shell—Planter's (7.0g/1oz.)
Walnuts— (3g/1/4 C.)
Peanut Butter—(See Tip Box pg. 155)

Dry, Grated Cheeses
Parmesan (.2g/1T. serving)
Romano (0g/1T. serving)

Spices, Herbs, Seasonings
Allspice (1.4/1tsp.)
Basil, dried crushed (.1g/1/4 tsp.)
Bay leaf (.1g/1 leaf)
Blackened Seasoning (0g/1/4 tsp.)
Bouillon granules
    Beef—1g/1tsp.
    Chicken—1g/1tsp.

Cajun Seasoning (0g/1/4 tsp.)
Caraway Seed (1.1g/1 tsp.)
Celery Salt (.6g/1tsp.)
Celery Seed (.9g/1tsp.)
Chili Powder (1.4g/1 tsp.)
Chives, chopped and dried (.1/1T.)
Cinnamon (2.1g/1 tsp.)
Cloves, ground (1.3g/1tsp.)
Cocoa, unsweetened (3g/1T.)
Coriander, ground (.2g/1/4 tsp.)
Cumin, ground (.9g/1 tsp.)
Dillweed, dried (.6g/1 tsp.)
Dry Salad Dressing Mixes
    —Good Seasons Italian(1g/serv.)
    —Hidden Valley Ranch (2g/serv.)
    —Garlic and Herb(1g/serv.)
Fennel seed (1.1g/1 tsp.)
Garlic Powder (2.3g/1 tsp.)
Garlic Salt (.5g/1 tsp.)
Ginger, ground (1.3g/1 tsp.)
Italian Seasoning Blend (.6g/1tsp.)
Lemon Pepper Seasoning (1.5g/1 tsp.)
Liquid Smoke (0g/1/4 tsp.)
Marjoram, dried crushed (.4g/1 tsp.)
Mustard, dry (.3g/1 tsp.)
Nutmeg, ground (1.1g/1 tsp.)
Onion, dry minced (1.9/1 tsp.)
Onion Powder (2.4g/1 tsp. serving)
Onion Salt (.4g/1 tsp. serving)
Onion Soup Mix, Lipton Recipe Secrets (4g/1T.)
Orange Peel, grated (1.5g/1 T.)
Oregano, dried, leaves or ground (.5g/1 tsp.)
Paprika (1.2g/1 tsp.)

Parsley, dry (.2g/1 tsp.)
Pepper,
    Black (1.7g/1 tsp. serving)
    Red or Cayenne (1.0/1 tsp. serving)
    Peppercorns (1.9/1tsp.)
Pumpkin Pie Spice (1.2g/1 tsp.)
Rosemary, dried (.8g/1 tsp.)
Sage, ground (.4g/1 tsp.)
Salt (0g)
Seasoned Salt (0g/1/4 tsp)
Sesame Seeds (.4g/1/4 tsp.)
Taco Seasoning Mix, Lawry's (5g/1T.)
Tarragon leaves, crushed (.8g/1 tsp.)
Thyme, ground (.9g/1 tsp.)
Vanilla (3g/1 tsp.)

Miscellaneous (Cooking/Baking/Frying/Etc.)
Broth, canned
    —Beef (2g/1 C.)
    —Chicken (1g/1 C.)
Cooking Oil Spray (such as, Pam^{TM}) (0g/serving)
Cornstarch (7g/1T.)
Gelatin
    Plain, Knox (0g/1pkt.)
    Sugar-free mixes, all flavors (Jell-O brand label states 0g./serving; other brands list between <1g and 1g/serving)
Oil—Corn, Olive, Sesame, Vegetable (0g)
Orange marmelade, Smucker's (13g/1 T.)
Pork rinds—Plain, Barbecue, and/or Hot and Spicy (for snacking, or grinding for coating and breading)—(0g)

Sweetener
 —Equal (Blue)—(<1g/packet)
 —Sweet and Low (Pink)—(1g/packet)
Vinegar—cider, red wine, white distilled (0g)
Wines, cooking (Holland House brand)
 Red (1g/2 T.)
 Sherry (2g/2 T.)
 White (0g/2 T.)

The Freezer

We store our meats and cheeses that are not going to be used immediately in the freezer. To increase your convenience at meal preparation time, consider some of the following pre-preparation suggestions:

** <u>Purchase meats and poultry in the family-pack, or bulk sizes</u> (you'll save money, and you're sure to eventually eat all that you buy). Then, split the packages up into smaller, meal-sized bundles before you put it in the freezer.

**<u>Bulk hamburger will defrost faster</u> if pressed into hamburger patties. Make patties, place into freezer bags and then into freezer. Then, you can defrost as many patties as you need for burgers, or molding back together for a loaf, or frying for ground beef.

**<u>Make-ahead meatballs</u>—As you are preparing the hamburger, you may want to prepare a batch of basic meatballs. Find a basic meatball recipe in this book and add the egg, binding crumbs, and seasonings as called for. Shape into balls. Place meatballs on a cookie sheet, barely touching each other. Put into freezer and allow to freeze on sheet for 45 minutes to an hour, or until firm. (This will keep the meatballs from sticking together.) Remove from pan and place into freezer bags. At meal time, you can remove as many meatballs as are needed, defrost, and continue preparation according to recipe.

**<u>Slice steak or round steak into strips</u> for fajitas or stir-frys (you may choose to go ahead and place in marinade, then freeze)

**<u>Rinse roasts and place in freezer containers</u> with seasonings for Italian beef, Herbed Rump Roast, or Pot Roast.

** <u>Poultry pre-preparation</u>: Disjoint chicken wings, cut up, and discard tips to save time at meal time. Rinse whole chickens and discard neck and organ package. Slice chicken breasts into nugget-sized portions for chicken nuggets or into strips for fajitas or stir-fry (follow the freezing method as for meatballs above to keep nuggets and strips from sticking together).

**<u>Pork pre-preparation</u>—De-bone, trim fat, and cube pork steak for pork chow mein. Separate bulk pork steak or chop packages into meal-sized or even individual packages so that you can defrost only the amount of steaks/chops that you need. Press bulk sausage into patties, and freeze as you would hamburger patties. Pre-boil pork ribs, in preparation for grilling or broiling at a later time.

The time and effort invested in pre-preparation activities will result in the ability to pull from the freezer near meal time (when we are tired, frazzled, and not thrilled about cooking) a main dish that is one step closer to being done.

Safety Note: When handling any meat and poultry, a clean working environment is essential! Please wash all work surfaces, utensils, and your hands before any food preparation activities. If you are preparing a variety of meats and poultry at one time, make sure to wash everything between preparation activities to prevent contact between the meats to lower risks of cross-contamination. Keep meats in the refrigerator until you are actually working with them.

If a meat is already frozen, you <u>cannot</u> completely defrost and then re-freeze it. If the meat contains some bacteria, the thawing/ re-freezing process may allow the bacteria to multiply and get such a foothold that, if it is then not properly cooked, food poisoning is a very real danger. You can *slightly* defrost the meat (say chicken breasts) to the point where you can slice it with a sharp knife. Then, *immediately* package and return it to the freezer.

Please allow "Be Clean! Be Safe!" to be your "battle cry" when working in the kitchen. Your family will thank you.

The following list is a skeleton inventory to create any recipe found in this cookbook. Keep amounts on hand that fit your family (and freezer) size.

Meats (0g carbs/serving)

Beef—Ground or Hamburger
- Roast
  - —Arm, boneless
  - —Chuck pot
  - —Roll rump, boneless
  - —Round rump
  - —Stew meat chunks
- Steaks
  - —Cube
  - —Flank
  - —Porterhouse
  - —Round
  - —Sirloin
  - —Strip
  - —T-bone

—**Chicken**
- Breasts, boneless/skinless
- Pieces
- Quarters
- Wings
- Whole

—**Turkey**
- Breast

—**Pork**
- Bacon
- Canadian bacon
- Chops
- Cutlets
- Ground
- Ham (Boneless, fully cooked)
- Ham Steaks

Loin or Shoulder Roast
Ribs, country-style and boneless
Sausage,
   —bulk, pork and Italian
   —link, including Italian, Polish, Bratwursts
Side Pork (also known as "Hog Jowl")
Spareribs or Country-style ribs
Steak

—**Fish, shellfish**
Fillets—catfish, whiting, orange roughy, etc.
Scallops
Shrimp,
   —popcorn
   —shelled and deveined

—**Lunch Meats/Deli Meats**
Deli-style chicken breast
Deli-style turkey breast
Ham
Pepperoni
Salami, including thin-sliced hard

Cheese
Freeze any variety of your favorite firmer cheeses, shredded, sliced, or in block form, (i.e., Cheddar, Mozzarella, Swiss, Monterey Jack, Colby, Colby-Jack, Muenster, Brick, etc.)

Frozen Vegetables
Asparagus, spears (2.9g/4 spears) or cut (4g/2/3 C.)
Broccoli florets (4g/1 1/3 C.)
Cauliflower florets (4g/1 C.)
Green beans, cut or French-style (5g/2/3 C.)

Vegetable blends (See Tip Box for more ideas on Page 142.)
—Green Giant varieties:
    California (2g/3/4 C. serving)
    Heartland (2g/1C. serving)
    Manhattan (1g/1C. serving)
    Santa Fe (4g/3/4 C. serving)
    Seattle (2g/3/4 C. serving)
—Bird's Eye varieties:
    Broccoli Stirfry (5g/1 C.)
    Broccoli, Cauliflower, and Carrots (4g/1 C.)
    Broccoli, Red Pepper, Onions, Mushrooms (4g/1 C.)
    Pepper Stir-Fry (5g/1 C.)
Fruit—Rhubarb (5g/1 C.)

The Refrigerator

You will want to keep several items on hand at all times since they seem to be used all the time. To minimize spoilage, we purchase fresh vegetables (that cannot be frozen) on a weekly basis. We've found that the dairy items that we use tend to have a fairly long refrigerator life, usually up to two weeks—if they aren't consumed by then! Here then is a basic refrigerator inventory to aid you in convenient recipe preparation:

Beverages
Flavored Waters (0g/serving)
Diet Soda (0g/serving)
(Mixes, Teas, and Coffee are listed under Pantry section)

Dairy
Butter (you can keep extra in the freezer) (0g/4oz. stick)
Cheeses pulled from freezer on as-needed basis (usually .91g. [<1g.] to 1g/oz.)
Brie cheese (.1g/1oz)

Cottage Cheese (4g/1/2 C.)
Cream cheese (<1g [approx. .91g]/oz.)
Heavy whipping cream (.4g/T., or 6.6g/1 C.)
Sour cream (1.22g/2T., or 9.8g/1 C.)

Eggs—(.6g/1 whole large egg)

Sauces, Seasonings, Condiments
For a complete listing of suggested dressings, marinades, and sauces please refer to the Salads and Dressings, Marinade Tip Box on page 76, or Sauces sections of this book. However, there are some items that will be "automatic" standards of your refrigerator inventory:
—Barbecue Sauce (See Tip Box pg. 150)
—Bottled Salad Dressing (See Tip Box on pg. 63)
    Caesar Dressing (2g/2 T.)
    Kraft Cucumber Ranch Dressing (2g/2 T.)
—Enchilada Sauce, Chi-Chi's or Old El Paso (3g/1/4 C.)
—Horseradish (0g/1 tsp.)
—Hot Sauce (Tabasco) (0g./1 tsp.)
—Lemon or lime juice (0g/1 tsp.—ReaLemon Brand)
—Marinades (See Tip Box pg. 76)
    Lawry's Mesquite with Lime
    Golden Dipt Southwest-Style Marinade
—Mayonnaise (0g/1 T.) Make sure that you purchase *real* mayonnaise, not salad dressing (such as Miracle Whip^{TM}). Also, do not buy low-fat or reduced-fat products, as these products will contain carbohydrates.
—Mustard,
    prepared (0g/1 tsp.)
    Dijon (<1g/1 tsp.)
—Pizza Sauce, Contadina (4g/1/4 C.)
—Salsa, Chi-Chi's or Old El Paso Homestyle (1g/2 T.)

—Soy Sauce, Kikkoman (0g/1 T.)
—Taco Sauce, Chi-Chi's or Old El Paso (1g/1 T.)
—Worcestershire Sauce, French's (<1g/1tsp.)

Fresh Vegetables
Asparagus, spears (2.6g/4 spears)
Avocados (12g/1 medium, 8oz.)
Broccoli (2.3g/1/2 C. chopped)
Cabbage—Green (1.9g/1/2 C. shredded)
           —Red (2.1g/1/2 C. shredded)
Carrots (7.3g/whole 7 1/2" long or, 5.6g/1/2 C. shredded)
Cauliflower (2.6g/1/2 C. 1"pieces)
Celery (2.2g/1/2 C. diced)
Cucumbers (8.3g/whole 8 1/4"long, or 1.4g/1/2 C. sliced)
Garlic cloves (1g/clove)
Lettuce—iceberg (11.3g/6" diameter head)
           —romaine (.7g/1/2 C. shredded)
Mushrooms (1.6g/1/2 C. raw pieces)
Okra (3.8g/1/2 C. sliced)
Onions—Green (3.7g/1/2 C. chopped
           —Red, White, Yellow (6.9 C./1/2 C. chopped)
Peppers, Green and Red Bell (3.2g/1/2 C. chopped)
Radishes, red (2.1g/1/2 C. sliced) and daikon (1.3g/1/2 C. sliced)
<u>Salad Blends,</u> (each with 3-4g/3 1/2 oz. serving):
    American
    European
    Spinach
    Caesar blend
Spinach leaves (1g/1/2 C. raw chopped)
Summer squash (2.75g/1/2 C. sliced)
Zucchini (1.9g/1/2 C. sliced)

Sample Menus

A comment that keeps re-occurring as we talk to people about the low-carbohydrate lifestyle is, "Yes, but how do you pull a meal together? I just get weary of trying to figure out what to fix." Space restrictions in this book prevent us from including all of the numerous menus that we have thought of, but in the following pages, we have included two weeks of dinner menus that our families have enjoyed, and that probably will "cost" you around 10-12 grams of carbohydrates total—and that's if you really stuff yourself. In the months to come, we hope to pull together a book of nothing but menus and their accompanying grocery lists to further aid you in creating easy, tasty, low-carbohydrate meals that you and your family will enjoy. But, for now we hope that the following examples will get you started and spark your creativity to pull together your own wonderful meals.

1. Broiled Chicken Wings
   Lettuce Salad with Toppings
   Cucumber-Ranch Dressing
   Deviled Eggs

2. Fajitas—(Beef, Chicken, and/or Shrimp)
   Toppings—Sour cream, Cheddar cheese, Black olives, taco sauce
   Guacamole

3. Pork Chops (Broiled, Fried, or Grilled)
   Classic Green Beans
   Cauliflower "Potato" Salad

4. Hamburgers or Cheeseburgers (Fried, Broiled, or Grilled)
   Relish Tray—Dill Pickles, Banana Peppers, and Olives
   Lettuce Salad with (small amount) Sweet Onions
   Peppercorn Ranch Dressing

5. Fried Fish Fillets
   Creamy Coleslaw
   Fried Vegetable Tray— zucchini slices, mushrooms, okra

6. Whole Baked Chicken
   Green Beans Amandine
   Wilted Lettuce Salad

7. Bacon-Wrapped Bratwursts
   Green Pepper/Onion Stirfry
   Spinach Salad

8. Meatloaf
   Broccoli, Cauliflower, and Carrot Vegetable Blend
       (Bird's Eye or Green Giant, for example)
   Cheese Sauce for meatloaf or vegetables
   Gelatin Salad

9. Fried Chicken Nuggets
   Fried Cheese Sticks
   Stuffed Celery
   Relish Tray—Pickles, Peppers, Olives

10. Pork Chow Mein
    Bean Sprout Salad

11. Taco Burgers
    Toppings—Lettuce, Sour Cream, Black olives
    Make-a-Dip-in-a-Flash, using taco seasoning mix
    Vegetable dippers—Cucumber slices, green pepper wedges, broccoli/cauliflower florets

12. Grilled Chicken Salad (Grilled Breast with Marinade)
    Bed of Greens
    Dressing (Buttermilk Ranch or Caesar to compliment marinade)
    Hard-boiled egg wedges
    Shredded cheese

13. Grilled (Marinated) Pork Steaks
    Coleslaw (with vinegar dressing)
    Fried Zucchini Patties

14. Italian Beef
    Caesar Salad
    Marinated Mozzarella

To create your own menus, we suggest that you fill in the following menu "framework" to suit your tastes, schedule, and budget:

> Main Dish Entree (if this is a meal-in-itself entree or a complete meal salad, you're done!)
> Salad
> Vegetable
> Appetizer as a Side Dish (optional)

We did not list dessert options with each menu since you will probably be limiting yourself during the weight-loss phase of your program. Please add the dessert recipes found in this cookbook as they fit into your program to suit your needs.

Appetizers and Snacks

The urge to snack is often considered to be the greatest challenge of dieters. It used to be our biggest nightmare. What a joy low-carbohydrate dining has been! Now, if truly hungry, we head straight to the kitchen with no fear or guilt tagging along behind us, and grab a bite of something to satisfy and sustain us. The trick to successful snacking is to have appropriate foods available to grab in a hurry—especially if there are high-carb. foods lurking in your kitchen.

We try to keep containers of the following foods (in addition to the recipes suggested in this section) in the refrigerator on-hand and available for the whole family:

- Fun Gelatin Squares (e.g., "Jell-o Jigglers^{TM}")
- A variety of cheese chunks and slices
- Chunks or slices of salami or other deli-meats
- Hard-boiled eggs (our kids love to peel and eat, with salt and pepper)

Also to be kept in the pantry, but always handy for quick-grab snacking:

- Pork rinds for munching or dipping
- Almonds (some flavors are O.K--such as smoked or barbecue)
- Pistachios and Macadamia nuts

A small sample of any one of these is usually enough to take the edge off our hunger without starting a carbohydrate binge like we used to experience before.

You may also consider the use of appetizers as a type of side dish to accompany your main entree as well as a snack, party fare, or the first course of a grand meal. Enjoy!

Barbecue-Sauced Meatballs

Carbs/serving: 1.21g/meatball

1 beaten egg	1/2 tsp. ground sage
2 T. water	1 lb. lean ground beef
3/4 C. pork rind crumbs	6 T. Hunt's Light barbecue sauce**
2 T. green onion,	2 T. orange marmalade,
finely chopped	*(optional)*
1/2 tsp. salt	Oil for frying

In a large bowl, combine egg and water. Stir in pork rind crumbs, onion, salt, and sage. Add meat and mix well. Shape into 36 or 48 meatballs. In a large skillet, fry meatballs in a small amount of oil until done. Remove to a plate lined with paper towels to drain. In a 2-quart saucepan combine barbecue sauce and marmalade. Stir in drained meatballs. Cover and cook meatballs over medium heat for 2 to 3 minutes or until sauce is hot, stirring gently once. Yield: 36 to 48 meatballs.

**Tip: For even lower carbs, consider making and using the low-carb barbecue sauces found in the Sauces section of this book.

Stuffed mushrooms are a wonderful party appetizer or side dish to accompany your meat entree. Here are just four suggestions, but you can let your imagination roam and see what tasty concoctions you can invent.

Basic Stuffed Mushrooms

Carbs/serving: 1g./mushroom (any variation)

24 large fresh mushroom, 1 1/2 to 2" in diameter

1/4 C. green onion, *chopped*	1/4 C. butter
1 clove garlic, *minced*	2 T. pork rind crumbs (See Tip box on page 72)

Use the Basic Stuffed Mushrooms ingredients for each of the following variations:

Sausage-Stuffed Mushrooms

Carbs/serving: .99g./mushroom

1/2 lb. bulk Italian sausage, *crumbled, fried, and drained*
2 T. Parmesan cheese, *grated*

Pepperoni-Stuffed Mushrooms

Carbs/serving: .93g./mushroom

1/4 C. pepperoni, *chopped*   1/2 C. mozzarella cheese, *shredded*

Ham-Stuffed Mushrooms

Carbs/serving: 1.03g./mushroom

1/4 C. ham, *finely chopped*   2 T. pecans, *chopped*

Seafood-Stuffed Mushrooms

Carbs/serving: 1.10g./mushroom

1 (3 oz.) pkg. cream cheese, *softened*	1/2 tsp. Worcestershire sauce
2 T. finely chopped pecans	1/4 tsp. salt
1/2 tsp. dried dillweed	Dash hot pepper sauce

1 (6 1/2) oz. can tuna, *drained* or 1 (6oz.) can crabmeat, *rinsed and drained*

For any variation of stuffed mushroom: Wash and drain mushrooms. Remove stems. Reserve caps. Chop enough stems to make 1 cup. In a medium saucepan, cook stems, onion, and garlic in butter until golden. Stir in remaining ingredients of chosen variation (For example, for Sausage variation, stir in fried sausage, and Parmesan cheese). Spoon mixture into mushroom caps. Arrange mushrooms in a baking pan. Bake in a 425° oven 8 to 10 minutes or until heated through. Makes 24.

Chili con Queso

Carbs/serving: .46g. /T.

1 T. butter	Dash bottled hot pepper sauce
1 C. heavy cream	1/2 C. salsa
1-8 oz. pkg. cheddar cheese, *shredded*	1 T. cornstarch
	1/4 C. cold water

In a saucepan, melt butter. Stir in cream and warm slowly. *Do not boil.* Stir in cheese until melted and smooth. Add salsa and hot pepper sauce (if desired). In a small bowl, combine cornstarch and cold water. Stir slowly into cream mixture. Continue cooking and stirring until mixture is thickened and hot throughout. Serve with fresh green pepper slices or pork rinds, or may be spooned over meatballs. Yield: Approx. 1 3/4 cups.

Salsa Dip

Carbs/serving: 2.3 g

1-8oz. pkg. cream cheese, *softened*	1 C. Salsa
1 C. Cheddar Cheese, *shredded*	1 C. Sour Cream

Preheat oven to 350°. Layer ingredients in an oven-proof glass bowl, in the following order: Spread cream cheese evenly over bottom of bowl, then salsa, and finally cheddar cheese on top. Warm in oven until cheddar cheese is melted and dip is hot throughout. Remove from oven and dollop sour cream over top of melted cheddar, then carefully spread sour cream evenly over top of dip. Serve warm with vegetable dippers or pork rinds. Yield: 16 servings.

To Prepare Salsa Dip in the Microwave: Follow instructions as above, but microwave on high (100%) for about 3 minutes, or until cheeses are melted and dip is hot throughout.

Guacamole

Carbs/Serving: .87/T.

2 medium avocados
1/4 C. onion, *chopped*
1-8 oz. pkg. cream cheese
1/2 tsp. salt

1 tsp. lemon or lime juice
1/2 tsp. Tabasco or hot sauce
(or to taste)

Cut avocados in half around pit; <u>*don't peel*</u>. Twist (like you would a peach) to separate the halves. Pry out the pit, and scoop out the meat of the avocado down to the rind. (This method is less messy and wasteful than trying to peel and slice the avocado). Mash avocado in a medium bowl. Add onion, cream cheese, lemon or lime juice, hot sauce, and salt. Mix well. Serve with vegetable dippers or pork rinds. Guacamole can also be served with any Mexican dish that you prepare, almost as a mini side-dish. Yield: Approx. 2 1/4 C. (or 40T.)

Spicy Cheese Dip for Vegetables

Carbs/serving: .66g

1 C. mayonnaise
4 tsp. mustard
4 tsp. dry mustard

1 1/2 C. cottage cheese
2 tsp. lemon juice
4 tsp. horseradish

Combine all ingredients; blend well. Chill. Serve with "legal" vegetable dippers. Yield: 20 servings.

Make-a-Dip-in-a-Flash

Carbs/serving: 1.73g

1-16oz. carton dairy sour cream
1 pkg. dry salad dressing mix (any Good Seasons Dressing Mix flavors, Hidden Valley Ranch Mix, etc.)
<u>or</u> 2 T. dry taco seasoning mix
<u>or</u> 2 T. dry onion and soup mix.

Stir sour cream and (dressing, seasoning, or soup mix) together well. Chill at least 2 hours to allow flavors to develop. Serve with vegetable dippers (green pepper slices, celery sticks, cucumber slices) or pork rinds. Yield: 16 servings.

Note: You can adjust the strength of your seasonings from milder to "wilder" by adding more or less seasoning mix. Be careful, though, as the taste strength of the dip will grow as the dip "rests" and "matures".

Be creative!! With a change in seasonings, you can create a complimentary dip and veggie side dish to go with any dinner. Serving a Mexican dish? Use taco seasoning. Italian? Use an Italian Dressing or Garlic and Herb blend. Of course, Ranch goes well with anything "American".

Cheese balls are a great invention! Wonderful for party fare, of course, they can also be kept on hand for instant snacking or a somewhat unusual side dish for dinner. Instead of 1 large cheese ball, you can shape walnut-sized cheese balls for individual servings (rolling each small cheese ball in its own particular coating). Add some fresh vegetables for a foundation, and, presto! instant snack or side dish. For the true cream cheese/cheese lover, these mini cheese balls are glorious just by themselves.

Party Cheese Ball

Carbs/serving: 1.36g

1 (8 oz.) pkg. cream cheese
2 C. cheddar cheese, *shredded*
1/4 C. green onion, *chopped*
2 tsp. Worcestershire sauce
1 T. lemon juice
1/3 to 1/2 C. pecans, *chopped*
(optional)

Mix softened cheese well, add other ingredients *except nuts*, chill and shape into ball. Roll in chopped nuts, if desired. Serve with green pepper wedges, celery sticks for stuffing, or spread over cucumber slices. Yield: 16 servings

Ham and Cheese Ball

Carbs/serving: 1.76g

1 (8 oz.) pkg. cream cheese, *softened*
2 C. Swiss cheese, *shredded*
1/4 C. green onion, *chopped*
2 T. heavy whipping cream
1 T. lemon juice
1 (3 oz.) can deviled ham,
or 1 (2.5oz.) pkg. thin-sliced ham, *shredded*
1/3 to 1/2 C. chopped pecans
(optional)

Mix softened cheese well, add other ingredients *except nuts*, chill and shape into ball. Roll in chopped nuts if desired. Serve alone or with green pepper slices. Yield: 16 servings.

Beefy Cheese Ball

Carbs/serving: .67g

1 (2 1/2 oz.) jar Armour Star Sliced Dried Beef, *rinsed and finely chopped*
1/4 C. sour cream
1/4 C. Parmesan Cheese, *grated*
1 (8oz.) pkg. cream cheese, *softened*
1 tsp. Prepared horseradish

Combine 1/4 cup dried beef, sour cream, cream cheese, Parmesan cheese, and horseradish. Blend thoroughly. Refrigerate 15 minutes. Form ball and roll in remaining dried beef. Chill. Serve with green pepper wedges or celery sticks. Yield: 16 servings.

Cheesy Bacon Cheese Ball

Carbs/serving: 1.25g

2-(8oz.) pkgs. cream cheese
2 T. onion, *chopped*
2 tsp. Worcestershire Sauce
1 tsp. lemon juice
8 oz. cheddar cheese, *shredded*
6 slices bacon, *fried and crumbled*

Soften cream cheese in small mixing bowl. Stir in onion, worcestershire, lemon juice, 1 cup cheddar cheese and bacon crumbles. Mix well. (*I usually use my hands at this point.*) Shape into a ball and coat evenly with remaining cheddar cheese. Refrigerate until ready to serve. Place on serving platter with vegetable dippers. Yield: 16 servings.

Appetizer Pie

Carbs/serving: 1.32g

1 (8-oz.) pkg. cream cheese
2 T. cream
1 pkg. dried beef, *shredded*
2 T. instant minced onion
2 T. minced green pepper
1/8 tsp. pepper
1/2 C. sour cream
1/4 C. coarsely chopped nuts

Have cream cheese at room temperature. Blend cheese with cream; stir in beef, onion, green pepper, pepper and sour cream. Blend well. Spoon into 8" glass pie plate or small shallow baking dish. Sprinkle with nuts. Bake at 350° for 15 minutes. Serve hot with vegetable dippers. Yield: 16 servings.

Buttermilk-Ranch Chicken Spread

Carbs/serving: 1.2g/T.

3 T. mayonnaise
2 T. dairy sour cream
2 T. buttermilk-ranch dressing mix
2 T. finely chopped nuts *(optional)*
1/2 C. cooked chicken, *finely chopped*
Green pepper wedges or deli-sliced chicken or turkey breast

In a medium mixing bowl combine mayonnaise, sour cream, and dry dressing mix. Mix until smooth. Stir in chopped nuts and chicken. Serve with green pepper wedges, or place 2 T. chicken spread on a slice of chicken or turkey breast and roll-up. Makes 2/3 cup spread (12 servings).

Ham Roll-Ups

Carbs/serving: 2.46g/roll-up

1 (16 oz.) pkg. sliced cooked ham *(16 slices)*
16 dill pickles spears, *well drained*
1 (8 oz.) pkg. cream cheese, *softened*

Spread each slice of ham with softened cream cheese. Drain pickle spears on paper towels to absorb extra juice. Place one pickle spear on the edge of each ham slice and roll up. Yield: 16 roll-ups.

Simple Summer Supper Idea!
(Say *that* 10 times fast!)
Chicken or turkey roll-ups
(made with the Buttermilk-Ranch Chicken Spread)
Ham Roll-ups
Deviled Eggs
Cheese Tray (slices of assorted cheeses)
Celery Sticks (with Sweetened Stuffing)
A generous plateful might add up to be only 10-12g. of carbs.

Salami Roll-Ups

Carbs/Serving: .29g/roll-up

1/2 lb. hard salami, *sliced thin (32 slices)*
1 (8oz.) pkg. cream cheese, *softened*
4-6 pepperoncini peppers, *seeded and chopped*

In a small bowl, combine cream cheese and chopped peppers. Spread cream cheese mixture across center of salami slices. Roll up jelly-roll fashion. Yield: 32 roll-ups.

Marinated Cheese and Olives

Carbs/serving: .98g

1 lb. cheese*, *your choice*	1 clove garlic, *minced*
2 oz. pepperoni or salami	1/4 tsp. fennel seed
1/4 C. olive oil or salad oil	1/4 tsp. pepper
2 T. lemon juice	1 (6 oz.) can pitted ripe olives, *drained*

Cut cheese and pepperoni or salami into 1/2" pieces. In a bowl combine next 5 ingredients. Stir in cheese, pepperoni or salami, and olives. Cover and chill up to 3 days, stirring occasionally. Let stand 30 minutes at room temperature before serving. Serve with toothpicks. Makes about 4 cups (16 servings).

*For example: Cheddar, Colby, Muenster, Monterey Jack, Mozzarella, Edam, Gouda, or a combination of cheeses.

Marinated Mozzarella

Carbs/serving: 1.3g

1 lb. Mozzarella cheese, *cut into thin 2" squares*	1 tsp. onion powder
	1 tsp. garlic powder
1/4 C. olive oil	1/4 tsp. ground black pepper
2 T. parsley, *finely chopped*	1 tsp. dried oregano leaves, *crushed*

Place cheese in a single layer in a 9x13" pan. In a small bowl, whisk next 6 ingredients. Pour oil mixture over cheese. Cover and refrigerate 8 hours or overnight to allow flavors to blend, turning slices occasionally. Yield: 16 servings.

Oven-Roasted Chili Brie

Carbs/serving: .55g

1 tsp. chili powder	1 pkt. sweetener
1/2 tsp. dry ground mustard	1 wheel Brie cheese (8oz)
1/2 tsp. garlic powder	1 T. softened butter

Preheat oven to 350°. Combine spices and sweetener; set aside. Spread butter in an oven-proof glass bowl; sprinkle lightly with spice mixture. Remove rind from Brie and place in bowl. Sprinkle Brie with remaining spice. Bake in oven 20-30 minutes or until melted and hot throughout. Serve with vegetable dippers. (We also like to eat this on a plate, plain, with a fork). Yield: 8 servings.

Fried Cheese Sticks

Carbs/serving: 1.5g

1 lb. whole mozzarella cheese*	1 tsp. onion powder
3 eggs, *beaten*	1/2 tsp. garlic powder
2 C. crushed pork rind crumbs (See Tip box on page 72)	

Cut mozzarella cheese into sticks approximately 3"x 1/2" thick. Allow to "rest" in freezer for 30 minutes prior to frying. Combine crushed pork rind crumbs, onion powder, and garlic powder in a small bowl and set aside. Put beaten eggs in another small bowl. Dip chilled cheese sticks in beaten egg, and then in coating mix until thoroughly and evenly coated. Meanwhile, heat oil in a heavy skillet just large enough to allow for 2 inches. When oil is hot, fry a few cheese sticks at a time to a golden brown. Drain on paper towels. Repeat until all cheese has been fried. Yield: 12 cheese sticks. (Serve with Contadina Pizza Sauce for dipping--1/4 cup adds a mere 4 grams of carbs.) (This also works well with cheddar cheese, too.)

Barbecued Chicken-Little "Legs"

Carbs/serving: .17/piece

3 lb. chicken wings (15-18 wings)
1/2 C. salad oil
1/2 C. lemon juice
1 clove of garlic, *crushed*
1 tsp. salt
1/8 tsp. pepper
1/2 C. pimento-stuffed olives, *chopped*

Cut wings at both joints; discard tips. Combine disjointed wing pieces with remaining ingredients. Marinate for several hours or overnight in refrigerator, stirring occasionally. Arrange wing pieces on rack in shallow roasting pan. Bake in 375° oven for 30 to 35 minutes or until crisp and browned. Spoon marinade over wings several times during baking time. Yield: 30-36 wing pieces

Buffalo Chicken Wings

Carbs/serving: 0g./piece

2 1/2 lbs. (12 to 15) chicken wings
1/4 C. Red Hot sauce (or more to taste)
1/2 C. butter, melted

Split wings at each joint and discard tips; pat dry. Deep fry at 400° (high) for 12 minutes or until completely cooked and crispy; drain. (Or, oven bake on a rack in a roasting pan at 425° for 15-20 minutes; turn halfway through cooking time.) Combine hot sauce and butter. Toss wings in sauce to coat. Makes 24 to 30 pieces.

Sweetened Stuffing for Celery Sticks
Carbs/serving: 1.37g/celery stick
1 (8 oz.) pkg. cream cheese, *softened*
Sweetener to equal 1/4 cup sugar (See Tip Box on page 48)
1 tsp. cinnamon *or* pumpkin pie spice
Approximately 24 celery sticks, 3-4" long

Combine cream cheese, sweetener, and the spice of your choice. Mix well. With a butter knife, fill the cavity of each celery rib. Will fill approximately 24 3" celery sticks. Keep refrigerated until ready to serve.

Fun Gelatin Squares
Carbs/serving: 0g*
4 pkgs (4 1/2-cup serving size) sugar-free gelatin, *any flavor*
or
2 pkgs (8 1/2-cup serving size) sugar-free gelatin, *any flavor*
2 1/2 C. boiling water

Mix gelatin with hot water until completely dissolved and blended. Pour into 9x13" pan (or smaller dish for thicker gelatin squares). Refrigerate until set--about 3 to 4 hours. Cut into squares. Keep refrigerated until serving time. (We try to keep these on hand in the refrigerator in a plastic-lidded container for quick snacking). Yield: 16 servings.

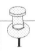

**Note: All sugar-free gelatin mixes are not created equal. Jell-O™ Brand states that it has 0g/serving, while other "off-brands" state having <1(which is usually in the range of .5-.9g), and still others state 1g/serving. So, be aware of your product's actual count before you allow yourself unlimited munching!

Beverages

Specialized beverages on a low-carbohydrate eating plan present their own challenges. Obviously, milk and fruit juices are too "expensive" from a carb-budget point of view, and almost all standard beverage recipes include some form of sugar. Even an attempt to lessen the carbohydrate load still results in the need to use quite a bit of artificial sweeteners, which may be a concern for those individuals who are hyper-sensitive to any sweetening agents.

During the weight-loss phase of your eating plan you will probably, like us, choose to save your carbohydrates for "real food"—that is, something that you can chew. Speaking from personal experience, we've found that it's difficult to have only one cup of eggnog or punch, and even if we've been able to reduce the carb count to only 4 or 5g. per cup, we could quite easily consume an entire day's carb "budget" in one sitting. For this reason, we've opted to save these beverages (and their recipes) for the maintenance phase of our eating lifestyle.

However, plain water (which we need plenty of, by the way, to wash away burnt fat remnants), diet sodas, tea, and coffee can become rather monotonous. There is good news! With a little imagination, you *can* widen the variety of your beverages. Following is a list of some ready-made beverages or beverage mixes, etc. with few to no carbs which you might want to incorporate into your diet:

Flavored Waters
Wal-Mart carries Clean and Clear™ in a wide variety of

flavors—the label states 0g./serving.

Schnuck's Stores carry Schnuck's Brand Naturally Flavored Spring Waters™—again, the label states 0g./serving.

Beverage Mixes

Country Time™ now has a new line of sugar-free drink mixes to go along with their sugar-free Lemonade and Pink Lemonade mixes. Give their sugar-free Lem N Berry Sippers™ (Strawberry Lemonade) a try. The label states 0g/serving.

Crystal Light™ has always had a wide variety of sugar-free beverage mixes that are delicious and convenient. They now have a new line of tropical flavors and flavored teas. You need to read the labels, though. Some flavors list 0g/serving, and others state <1g/serving (again, which can mean anywhere from .5-.9g/serving).

Flavored Teas

Lipton™ now has a line of sugar-free instant flavored teas (Raspberry, Peach, and Lemon) that are tasty and convenient, but they will cost 1g/serving.

Celestial Seasonings™ has long offered a fantastic variety of herbal teas. (Please try the new Caribbean Kiwi Peach™. It is wonderful!) These teas are most likely caffeine free, although there are some flavors that do have caffeine. You have to take the time to brew them, but you have full control of the sweetener you add, and therefore, your carb count. As is, with no sweeteners added, these teas weigh in at 0g/serving.

Flavored Coffees

Kroger's™ and Schnuck's™, as well as Gloria Jean's™ and other gourmet coffee shops offer a huge assortment of flavored coffee beans that you can grind and brew fresh. (And, if you look sharp, there are decaffeinated flavors as well.) When we want to treat ourselves to something simple yet elegant, we brew a pot of an interesting flavor ("Danish Pastry" by Millstone from Kroger's is to die for!), add sweetener and cream to taste, and top off with a small dollop of whipped cream and a sprinkle of cinnamon. This wonderful dessert coffee (we call it a "Pseudo-Cappuccino") can be just the right ending to a dinner party with friends, a quiet dinner for two, or a reward for weary parents after the children are finally asleep. Be careful not to get too hooked, though! Each cup will cost you between 2-3g of carbs, depending upon the amount of sweetener and cream you use. (A cup of black coffee will cost approximately .8g.)

Diet Sodas

Just a brief mention, please! There is more to the diet soda world than diet colas, rootbeer, or lemon-lime varieties. If you would like a change of pace from the standard variety, don't forget that Shasta™ carries a variety of flavors (from ginger ale to grapefruit) that could also be served in lieu of a sugary party punch. Each label states 0g/serving.

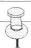

Please be a label reader! (We hope that you will not weary of us saying this. But, it is almost a mantra-chant, it is so important.)

A product might be labelled "sugar-free" and yet contain some natural sugars, sugar derivatives, or some form of carbohydrates deep within the list of ingredients. (Look for the "-oses"—fructose, lactose, dextrose, sucrose, maltose, glucose). Even though the label may state 0g/serving, it may in actuality contain from .1-.4g/serving. For example, heavy whipping cream is generally labelled as 0g/T. and one may think that cream therefore is a free and unlimited food. But, one cup of cream (16 T.) has 6.6g of carbs! Doing the math, 6.6 divided by 16 equals .41g/T. If a label states that there is <1g./serving, it means that it can contain from .5-.9g/serving, and the manufacturer chose not to round up to 1g. This information is not intended to upset, discourage, or create carbohydrate paranoia, but to enlighten and arm you with the information you need to make the best choices possible, and to make you aware of what you're eating so that you can be successful with this eating lifestyle that you have chosen. Our best advice is to eat and drink a wide variety of foods and beverages. We've found that not getting into a rut somehow better satisfies our appetite, both physically and psychologically. We seem to get by on less food and drink with no feelings of deprivation. We hope it works the same way for you!

Salads and Dressings

Salads need not be a boring fare of only cut lettuce leaves and a drizzle of salad dressing. With just a little time and imagination, you can create an attractive, tasty, and relatively low-carbohydrate accompaniment to your main meat entree. Or, you may choose to select one of the meal-in-itself recipes (such as Taco Salad or Fried Chicken Salad) on an evening when time is short or the weather is hot for a quick, yet satisfying dinner. We have had to train ourselves (and our families) to not be afraid when we set only one, two, or three bowls of food on the table. Through experience with this way of eating, we have learned that though sometimes the table may appear to be bare, our appetites and our tummies will be totally satisfied at the meal's end.

Have you tried the salad mixes in the produce section of your grocery store? There are a variety of blends that are a little more pricey than purchasing a head of lettuce, but will save you time. For many of the following recipes that call for cut lettuces (iceberg or romaine) or shredded cabbage, you may choose to substitute a bag of salad or coleslaw blend.

We entitled this salad "The Salad of a Million Faces" as a catchy name for the traditional cut lettuce salad and toppings. But, you can go in so many directions that your salad might not ever be the same way twice, and therefore you can create an almost endless variety. Think about the main dish that you are serving, and try to compliment those flavors with your choice of salad "fixin's". The number of carbs/serving will fluctuate with your choices, but should remain within a reasonable range. We've also found that preparing a salad this way (as a side dish on the table) for some reason seems to be more satisfying to our family than if we present all of the ingredients salad bar fashion and have everyone make their own salad. Lastly, our own personal practice is to serve our salads on our dinner plates rather than in separate salad bowls. Everyone's plates are fuller and we don't seem to overload ourselves with larger portions to fill up the empty spaces.

"The Salad of a Million Faces"

Carbs/Serving: 4.04 to 5.78g (Will range according to your selection of ingredients)

1 pkg. salad mix, *your choice*:
    American
    European
    Spinach

Up to 1 C. of 1 or 2 of the following:
    radishes, red or daikon, *sliced or grated*
    fresh mushrooms, *sliced*
    cucumber, *peeled and sliced or chopped*

Up to 1/2 C. of 1 or 2 of the following:
    green bell pepper, *chopped*
    red bell pepper, *chopped*
    green onion, *chopped*
    olives, (green pimiento stuffed or ripe) *sliced or chopped*

Up to 1 C. of any of the following:
    shredded cheeses, such as: Cheddar, mozzarella, colby-jack, Swiss
    bacon, *crisp-fried and crumbled*

ham, *finely diced*
chicken, *cooked and cubed*
leftover roast, *thinly sliced or shredded*
1/4 C. to 1/2 C. Bottled dressing of your choice (See the Tip box later in this section for your best low-carb. choices)

In a large salad bowl, toss together salad greens and any other salad ingredients that you have chosen. Just before serving, pour dressing over salad and toss lightly. Serve well-chilled. Yield: 6 servings.

1-Minute Caesar Salad

Carbs/Serving: 3.65g.
4 C. romaine lettuce, *torn*
1/4 C. to 1/2 C. bottled Caesar Dressing
1/2 C. Parmesan Cheese

In a large salad bowl, place lettuce. Just before serving, toss lettuce with dressing and cheese. Yield: 4 servings.

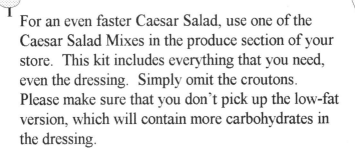

For an even faster Caesar Salad, use one of the Caesar Salad Mixes in the produce section of your store. This kit includes everything that you need, even the dressing. Simply omit the croutons. Please make sure that you don't pick up the low-fat version, which will contain more carbohydrates in the dressing.

Hearty Italian Salad

Carbs/Serving: 4.61g

4 C. iceberg lettuce, *torn*
4 C. Romaine lettuce, *torn*
1/2 C. grated Parmesan Cheese
1 small jar pimento, *chopped*
1 C. red onion, *sliced*
1 can artichoke hearts, *quartered (optional)*
2/3 C. oil
1/3 C. red wine vinegar
1 pkt. Sweetener
1 pkg. Good Seasons Italian Dressing mix

Combine first 6 ingredients. Mix vinegar, oil, sweetener, and dressing mix; stir until well blended. Pour over lettuce mixture; toss well. Refrigerate. Yield: 10 servings.

Layered Lettuce Salad

Carbs/Serving: 3.28g

1 small head lettuce, *torn into small pieces*
1 C. celery, <u>diced</u>
4 eggs, *hard boiled and sliced*
1/2 C. green pepper, *sliced*
1/2 C. green onion, *chopped fine*
8 slices bacon, *crisply fried and crumbled*
2 C. mayonnaise
2 pkts. Sweetener
1/2 C. Parmesan cheese, *grated*
4 oz. cheddar cheese, *shredded*

Tear lettuce up in bite size pieces and put in bottom of 9x13" glass dish. Layer rest of ingredients in the following order: celery, eggs, green pepper, onion, and finally bacon. In a small mixing bowl, combine mayonnaise, sweetener and Parmesan cheese; mix until well blended. Spread over top of salad as you would icing on a cake. Top with grated cheese. Cover and refrigerate from 8-12 hours. Do not stir until ready to serve. Then only toss lightly. Yield: 9 servings.

Wilted Salad

Carbs/Serving: 4.58g

5 slices bacon
6 C. lettuce or fresh spinach leaves, *torn*
3 hard-boiled eggs, *sliced (optional)*
Dressing:
2 T. bacon drippings (or, melted butter)
1/4 C. vinegar
1 tsp. onion powder
1 pkt. sweetener

To make dressing: In a small pan, fry the bacon until crisp, reserving 2 T. of the bacon drippings; remove bacon from pan and drain. When cool, crumble; set aside. Heat the reserved drippings and add the vinegar, onion powder and sweetener. Heat thoroughly, but do not boil. Add crumbled bacon back to dressing. In a large salad bowl, place salad greens. Just before serving, pour hot dressing over greens and toss quickly. If desired, garnish with hard-boiled egg slices. Serve immediately. Makes 4 servings.

Cole Slaw

Carbs/Serving: 4.66g.

1 medium head cabbage, *shredded*
For dressing:

1 C. vinegar	1 tsp. dry mustard
1 tsp. celery seed	1 tsp. onion powder
3/4 C. salad oil	Sweetener to equal 1 C. sugar (See Tip Box on page 48)

To make dressing: Mix together all dressing ingredients in a medium saucepan, except the Sweetener. Bring to a boil, then turn off heat. Stir in sweetener. In a large bowl, place shredded cabbage. Pour hot dressing over slaw. Cover bowl tightly. Refrigerate overnight to allow flavors to develop. (Will stay good in refrigerator for 1 week). Yield: 16 servings.

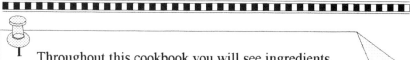

Throughout this cookbook you will see ingredients listed as "Sweetener equal to (amount) sugar". This is listed in this way to allow you to choose what type of sweetener you prefer. Aspartame sweeteners (blue packets) taste more like sugar to us than Sweet 'n Low™ -type sweeteners (pink packets), but you will probably need to use more blue packets than pink—especially when cooking or baking with high heat or for longer periods of time. "Pink" sweeteners holds up a bit better under heat than "blue" sweeteners, but tend to have a little more bitter taste. So, the choice is yours. For your convenience, we've listed a sweetener conversion chart below. Even though both "blue" and "pink" sweetener boxes listed the very same conversion charts, we still maintain that you won't need to use as many pink packets (you can almost cut it in half). Always refer to the charts or suggestions listed on the actual product that you are using, and ultimately let your taste buds be your guide.

Sweetener	Sugar
1 packet	2 teaspoons
6 packets	1/4 cup
8 packets	1/3 cup
12 packets	1/2 cup
16 packets	2/3 cup
18 packets	3/4 cup
24 packets	1 cup

Creamy Coleslaw

Carbs/Serving: 4.70g.

6 C. cabbage, *shredded*
1/2 C. carrot, *grated*
1 C. green pepper, *chopped fine*

Dressing:
1 C. mayonnaise
2 tsp. vinegar
1/8 tsp. Worcestershire sauce
1/4 C. green onions, *finely chopped*
1/4 tsp. salt
1/8 tsp. pepper
1 pkt. sweetener, or less to taste

In a large salad bowl, place cabbage, carrot, and green pepper; toss to combine. In a small bowl, mix together all dressing ingredients until well blended. Pour dressing over salad, toss lightly, and serve. Makes 8 servings.

Chinese Coleslaw

Carbs/Serving: 4.5g

1 (16oz.) pkg. coleslaw blend (found in the produce section of your store)
1/4 C. green onions, *chopped*
1/2 C. slivered almonds
For dressing:
3/4 C. oil
1/2 C. vinegar
Sweetener to equal 3/4 C. sugar
3 T. soy sauce

In a large bowl, mix together cabbage, onions, and almonds. In a small bowl, mix together all dressing ingredients. Mix well. Pour dressing over slaw. Let stand at least one hour before serving to allow flavors to develop. Yield: 12 servings.

Deb's Cucumbers

Carbs/Serving: 5.1g

2 medium cucumbers
salt
1 C. red onion, *sliced thin*
Dressing:
1 C. mayonnaise
1 tsp. apple cider vinegar
1 tsp. cream

Peel and slice cucumbers. Place in a large mixing bowl and sprinkle with salt. Cover with a lunch plate and weight down with a can or other heavy object to draw the juice. Put in refrigerator overnight. Remove plate and can. Drain juice, rinse, and drain well again. Add red onion slices. In a small bowl mix dressing ingredients in order to make a thick dressing.
Yield: 6 servings.
Note: You can skip the salting, and juice-drawing step if you are wanting to serve the salad immediately. But, if you prepare it ahead of time without this step be aware that the salad will become very watery, as will any leftovers.

Vinegar Cucumber Salad

Carbs/Serving: 3.84g

2 medium cucumbers, *peeled and sliced thin*
Salt ,pepper and onion powder to taste
Dressing:
1/4 C. oil
1/4 C. vinegar
Sweetener to equal 1/4 C. sugar

In a medium serving bowl, place cucumber slices; sprinkle with salt, pepper, and onion powder to taste. In a small bowl, mix together dressing ingredients until well blended. Pour dressing over salad before the oil and vinegar separate. Serve the salad well chilled. Yield: 6 servings.

Bean Sprout Salad

Carbs/Serving: 3.42g

6 C. romaine lettuce or fresh spinach leaves, *torn*
2 C. canned bean sprouts, *drained*
1/2 C. toasted slivered almonds

Dressing:

1/4 C. green onions, *finely chopped* 1/4 tsp. coriander
3 T. chopped parsley   1/2 tsp. ginger
1 T. soy sauce   2 T. mayonnaise
1/2 C. dairy sour cream   2 T. cream

In a large salad bowl, toss together all salad ingredients. In a small bowl, mix together all dressing ingredients until well blended. Just before serving, pour dressing over salad; toss lightly. Makes 10 servings.

Hot Green Bean Salad

Carbs/Serving: 5.22g

2 (14.5oz.) cans cut green beans, *drained*
3 slices bacon, *fried crisp and crumbled*

Dressing:

2 T. bacon drippings (or, melted butter)
1/4 C. vinegar
1 tsp. onion powder
1 pkt. sweetener

To make dressing: In a small pan, fry the bacon until crisp, reserving 2 T. of the bacon drippings; remove bacon from pan and drain. When cool, crumble; set aside. Heat the reserved drippings and add the vinegar, onion powder and sweetener. Heat thoroughly, but do not boil. Add crumbled bacon and beans back to dressing. Toss until beans are coated with dressing. Heat until green beans are hot throughout. Place in a serving bowl and serve warm. Makes 6 servings.

Summer Salad

Carbs/Serving: 3.3g
4 C. cauliflower florets
2 C. broccoli florets
1/2 C. small jar salad olives, *chopped*
1 pkt. Good Seasons Italian Dressing/ or Seven Seas Salad Dressing,
prepared according to packet directions

In a large salad bowl, combine chopped raw vegetables. Mix with olives. Add salad dressing to taste. Refrigerate. Yield: 12 servings.

St. Louis Salad

Carbs/Serving: 3.9g
6 C. broccoli florets
1 C. red onion, *sliced thin*
Dressing:
1 C. mayonnaise
Sweetener to equal 1/4 cup sugar or to taste

Combine in a large salad bowl the broccoli and onions. In a small bowl, combine the mayonnaise and sweetener; stir until well blended. Pour dressing over the salad and toss until salad is lightly coated. Serve well chilled. Yield: 12 servings.

Please give this next recipe a try! At first, we wrinkled our noses at the thought of a cauliflower substitute for potatoes, too. But, it really works! If you like this recipe, consider trying a cauliflower substitute for your family's favorite potato salad recipe. We think that you will be pleasantly surprised.

Cauliflower "Potato" Salad

Carbs/Serving: 4.11g

6 C. cauliflower florets
1/2 C. heavy cream
1/4 C. vinegar
1 egg, *beaten*
4 T. butter
3/4 tsp. celery seed
1/4 tsp. dry mustard

Sweetener to equal 1/3 C. sugar
1/4 C. onion
1/4 C. mayonnaise
3 hard-boiled eggs, *chopped*
6 slices bacon, *fried crisp, crumbled*
Paprika

In a large pan of boiling water, blanch cauliflower until florets are just fork-tender. Drain and rinse with cold water to stop the cooking process. Set aside. In a small saucepan, combine next 6 ingredients. Cook and stir over low heat until bubbly. Remove from heat; add sweetener, onion and mayonnaise. Cool. In serving bowl, combine cooked, cooled cauliflower, hard-boiled eggs, and bacon. Gently fold in dressing. Chill. Just before serving, sprinkle with paprika. Yield: 12 servings.

Cauliflower-Lettuce-Bacon Salad

Carbs/Serving: 3.37g

6 C. iceberg lettuce, *torn*
4 C. cauliflower florets
1 lb. bacon
1 1/2 C. mayonnaise
1/2 C. Parmesan cheese
Sweetener to equal 1/4 C. sugar

In a skillet, fry bacon. Drain, cool, and crumble. Set aside. In a large salad bowl, combine lettuce, cauliflower and bacon. To make dressing, combine mayonnaise, cheese, and sweetener. Gently fold dressing into salad. Chill until ready to serve. Yield: 12 servings.

Taco Salad

Carbs/Serving: 4.46g

4 C. iceberg lettuce, *torn*
1 (8 oz.) pkg. cheddar cheese, *shredded*
2 lb. ground beef, *browned and drained*
Salt, pepper and onion powder to taste
Sour cream
Taco sauce

Bring to the dinner table all ingredients in separate bowls. To assemble the salad, layer 1 cup lettuce, ground beef, cheese, sour cream (up to 2 T.) and taco sauce (up to 1T.) on each plate. Yield: 4 servings.

Note: If you or your family desires more taco seasoning, you may mix up to 4 tsps. of dry taco seasoning mix into the ground beef after it is browned and drained. This will add approximately 2 g. of carbs to each serving.

You can double this recipe and serve it as a complete meal. 2 helpings of this salad is very filling, and you've only eaten 8.92g of carbs for an entire dinner!

Fried Chicken Salad
(This is a meal in itself!)

Carbs/Serving: 6.71g

4 boneless skinless chicken breasts
2 eggs, *slightly beaten*
2-3 C. pork rind crumbs *(for breading)*
Oil for frying
4 C. iceberg lettuce, *torn*
4 hard-boiled eggs, *quartered*
1 (8 oz.) pkg. shredded cheese *(your choice)*
Kraft Cucumber Ranch Dressing

Cut chicken breasts into cubes or strips. Dip chicken pieces into egg and roll in pork rind crumbs. Heat oil in a deep skillet or deep-fat fryer to 400° (high). Fry chicken pieces until done (approximately 3-5 minutes each, depending on size of pieces). Drain on paper towels and allow to cool. To assemble the salad, place 1 cup of lettuce on each plate. Lay chicken pieces atop lettuce, and garnish with hard-boiled egg quarters. Drizzle up to 3 tablespoons of dressing over salad. Yield: 4 servings.

This is so easy, delicious, and filling. What really makes this salad so tasty is the dressing. But, watch how much you use: Each tablespoon will cost you 1g carb, which doesn't sound bad, but they can add up quickly.

Caesar Chicken Salad

Carbs/Serving: 2.4g.

4 boneless skinless chicken breasts
4 T. butter
1 T. oil
4 C. romaine lettuce
Parmesan cheese
Bottled Caesar Salad Dressing

Slice chicken breasts into strips. Melt butter in a skillet and add oil to prevent butter from burning. Fry chicken pieces in butter and oil until done (approximately 3-5 minutes). Remove from pan and allow to cool. To assemble salad, place 1 cup of lettuce on plate. Lay chicken pieces atop lettuce, drizzle with Caesar salad dressing (up to 3 tablespoons), and sprinkle with Parmesan cheese. Yield: 4 servings.

Hot Chicken Salad

Carbs/Serving: 3.08g

6 C. chicken, *cooked and chopped into small bites*
2 T. lemon juice
1/2 C. heavy cream
1 C. mayonnaise
3 tsp. chicken bouillon granules
2 C. celery
4 hard boiled eggs, *chopped*
2 tsp. onion powder

Topping:
1 C. cheddar cheese, *shredded*
1 (2oz.) pkg. slivered almonds

Preheat oven to 350°. Mix together first 8 ingredients. Spoon into buttered 9x13" baking pan. Bake in oven 15 minutes. Sprinkle cheese and almonds over top of casserole. Bake an additional 10-15 minutes or until cheese is melted and casserole is hot throughout. Yield: 12 servings.

Chinese Chicken Salad
Carbs/Serving: 4.10g
3 C. lettuce, *torn*
3 C. chicken, *cooked and chopped*
1/2 C. canned bamboo shoots, *drained*
1/2 C. carrots, *julienned*
1/4 C. green onions, *sliced diagonally*
1/2 C. red cabbage, *chopped*
Dressing:
3 1/2 T. soy sauce
2 T. vegetable oil
2 T. vinegar
2 pkts. sweetener, or to taste
1/2 tsp. each: garlic powder, black pepper, and sesame oil (optional)

In a small bowl, whisk together dressing ingredients; set aside. In large salad bowl, combine remaining salad ingredients. Just before serving, toss salad with dressing. Makes 6 servings.

Crunchy Chicken Salad
Carbs/Serving: 4.16g
6 C. cooked chicken, *cubed*
2 C. celery, *diced*
1 C. fresh mushrooms, *sliced*
1 (2oz.) pkg. pecan halves
4 slices bacon, *fried crisp and crumbled*
1 C. green onions, *sliced*
Dressing:
1/2 C. sour cream
3/4 C. mayonnaise
1 T. lemon juice

In a large bowl, toss together chicken, celery, and mushrooms. In a small bowl, combine dressing ingredients; mix together until well-blended. Pour dressing over salad and toss until moistened. Chill. Before serving, stir in pecans, bacon, and green onions. Yield: 8 servings.

Ham and Cheese Salad

Carbs/Serving: 3.37g

3 C. lettuce, *torn*
2 C. boiled or baked ham, *cubed*
3 hard-boiled eggs, *sliced*
1 (8oz.) pkg. Cheddar cheese, *shredded*

Dressing:
3/4 C. sour cream, *(or more as needed)*
3/4 C. mayonnaise, *(or more as needed)*
1/4 C. lemon juice
1/2 C. Parmesan cheese, *grated*
2 tsp. dried tarragon leaves, *crumbled (optional)*
1/2 tsp. salt
1/2 tsp. pepper
1/2 tsp. liquid red-pepper seasoning (Hot sauce)

Combine lettuce, ham, cheese, and eggs in a large bowl. Combine dressing ingredients in a small bowl; stir to mix well. Pour dressing over salad; toss well to blend. Yield: 6 servings.

Variation: Use 3 C. finely shredded cabbage instead of the lettuce and omit hard-boiled eggs.

Tuna Salad

Carbs/Serving: .85g

4 (6oz.) cans tuna fish, *drained*
1/2 C. celery, *chopped*
1/4 C. mayonnaise (or more as needed to reach consistency desired)
2 T. dill pickle relish
2 hard-boiled eggs, *chopped (optional)*

In a medium bowl, combine together all ingredients and mix until thoroughly blended. Serve salad well-chilled on lettuce leaves. Makes 4 servings.

Variation: This recipe can become a simple meat salad by substituting chicken (cooked and cubed), diced or ground ham, corned beef, or leftover roast for the tuna.

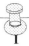

The following 3 recipes have been included in the Salads section, but you could also consider serving them as a light dessert as well.

Carrot-Pineapple Gelatin Salad
Carbs/Serving: 3.77g.
2 small (4-1/2 C. serving size) pkg. sugar-free orange gelatin
2 C. hot water
2 C. cold water
1 C. crushed pineapple, *drained*
1 C. carrots, *grated*

In a medium mixing bowl, prepare gelatin mix according to package directions. Place in the refrigerator until thickened. Fold in carrots and pineapple. Spoon into 9"x13" pan and chill in refrigerator until set. Yield: 12 servings.
Variation: Omit carrots and consider serving this as a dessert topped with a small dollop of whipped cream.

Strawberry and Rhubarb Salad Molds
Carbs/Serving: 2.05g.
3 C. hot water
1 (16oz.) pkg. frozen rhubarb
3 small (4-1/2 C. serving size) pkgs. sugar-free strawberry-flavored gelatin
Sweetener to equal 1/4 C. sugar

In a medium saucepan, heat water to boiling. Add rhubarb to hot water; cook for 3-5 minutes, or until rhubarb begins to soften. Dissolve gelatin and additional sweetener in hot water/rhubarb mixture. Pour into serving dish, or gelatin mold. Refrigerate until set. If using a mold, at serving time, dip mold briefly into warm water to loosen. Makes 10 servings.

Orange or Lime Fluff

Carbs/Serving: 3.99g

2 small (4-1/2 C. serving size) pkgs. sugar-free orange or lime gelatin
2 C. hot water
1 (8oz.) pkg. cream cheese, *softened*
1 C. crushed pineapple, *drained*
1 C. cream, *whipped to soft peaks*

Dissolve Jello in hot water. While still hot, mix in cream cheese. (You may want to use a mixer to get a smoother consistency). Refrigerate until gelatin begins to thicken. Add pineapple. Fold in whipped cream. Spoon into 9x13" pan. Chill until firm. Yield: 12 servings.

Variation: For a wider array of possibilities (and lower carbs), you can omit the pineapple and use any flavor of sugar-free gelatin mix that you desire. Without the pineapple, the carbs drop to 1.16g/serving.

While bottled salad dressings are convenient, homemade salad dressings are significantly lower in carbohydrates because you control all of the ingredients that are included. If you have the time you may wish to try some of the following recipes. You can then allow yourself to be more liberal when applying dressings to your salads.

Creamy Cucumber Dressing

Carbs/Serving: .28g/T.
1 1/2 C. cucumber, *peeled, seeded, chopped*
1 C. mayonnaise
1 T. cream
1 T. lemon juice
2 T. chives, chopped

Place ingredients in blender or food processor and blend until smooth. Keep covered in refrigerator. Yield: Approximately 1 1/2 cups (or 24T).

French Dressing

Carbs/Serving: .27g/T.
1 C. mayonnaise
3 T. lemon juice
2 T. chopped parsley
1 T. paprika
1 T. cream
1 pkt. sweetener, or to taste
1/2 tsp. dried tarragon leaves, crumbled
1/2 tsp. dry mustard

Blend ingredients together until well mixed, cover, and chill. Yield: Approximately 1 1/2 cups (or 24T.).

Parmesan Dressing

Carbs/Serving: .24g/T.
1 C. mayonnaise
1/3 C. Parmesan cheese, *grated*
1/4 C. chopped parsley
1/4 C. cream
2 T. lemon juice
1 tsp. dried basil leaves
1 tsp. dried marjoram leaves

Blend ingredients together, cover, and chill. Yield: Approximately 1 1/2 cups (or 24T.)

Creamy Italian Dressing

Carbs/Serving: .14g/T.

1 C. mayonnaise	1 clove garlic, *pressed*
3 T. cream	1/2 tsp. dried oregano leaves
2 T. cider vinegar	1 pkt. sweetener

Blend ingredients together, cover, and chill. Yield: Approximately 1 1/2 cups (or 24T).

Vinaigrette Dressing

Carbs/Serving: .16g/T.

4 pkts. sweetener	1 1/2 tsp. green olives, *chopped*
1 tsp. salt	1 1/2 tsp. parsley, *chopped*
1/2 tsp. leaf basil, *crumbled*	2 tsp. green onion, *chopped*
1/2 tsp. leaf oregano, *crumbled*	1/2 tsp. cayenne (red) pepper
1/4 tsp. dry mustard	2 C. vegetable oil
Pinch black pepper	1 hard-boiled egg, *chopped*
Pinch garlic powder	
1/2 C. red wine vinegar	

Combine first 8 ingredients in a large screw-top jar; shake well to mix. Add the olives and remaining ingredients to the jar; shake once again to mix well. Store in the refrigerator. Yield: Approximately 2 1/2 cups (or 40T.)

Theresa's Vinegar-Mustard Dressing

Carbs/Serving: .20g/T.

1/2 C. vinegar	Sweetener to equal 1/4 C. sugar
1 1/4 C. oil	1 T. prepared mustard

In a small jar with a screw-top lid, thoroughly combine all ingredients. Chill until ready to serve. Just before serving, mix or shake to recombine ingredients. Yield: Approximately 1 3/4 cups (or 28 T.)

Variation: Omit prepared mustard and substitute 1 tsp. celery seed.

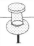

Your Guide to Bottled Salad Dressings

When time and inclination prevents you from making your own dressings, use the following guide to help you find the best carbohydrate "buys" in bottled dressings— which will typically be dressings with a creamy base. Do NOT buy low-fat or fat-free dressings as these can, for some products, almost double the amount of carbohydrates. The following is a partial list of dressings that we have scouted out which have a fairly low carb. count. But, don't consider this to be an exhaustive list; if you happen upon other flavors and brands at your local store, add them to your pantry list, and enjoy!

Kraft Brand—each with 1-2g/2T.

Bacon and Tomato   Zesty Garden (Kraft Salsa)
Buttermilk Ranch   Italian (Kraft Free)
Caesar   Peppercorn Ranch
Creamy Garlic   Ranch
Cucumber Ranch   Sour Cream and Onion

Seven Seas Brand—each with 1-2g/2T.

Creamy Caesar   Italian (Seven Seas Viva)
Creamy Italian   Ranch
Green Goddess   Red Wine Vinegar and Oil
Herb and Spices

Wishbone Brand—each with 1-2g/2T.

Italian (Wishbone Classic House)
Ranch   Sierra

Lawry's Brand

Creamy Caesar with Cracked Pepper (1g. carb/2T.)

Marie's

Parmesan (2g/2T.)

Brianna's

Homestyle Real French Vinaigrette (0g/2T.) (Excellent on hot vegetables and meat!)

Meaty Main Dishes

The heart of any low-carbohydrate program is the protein—that is, the meats, cheeses, and eggs that you can heartily and joyfully eat. We have included our families' favorite recipes—entrees that are delicious, yet convenient and affordable. When you prepare your meals, make sure that you are liberal with your main dish amounts. This will allow you to satisfy your appetite with the high protein/low carbohydrate foods that you need to lose weight and feel better. If our recipe sizes don't fit your family, please feel free to expand or reduce them accordingly.

Poultry

Broiled Lemon Pepper Chicken Wings
Carbs/Serving: 0g.
3 lb. chicken wings (15-18 wings)
Lemon Pepper Seasoning
1 stick butter (melted)

Rinse chicken wings; sprinkle with lemon pepper seasoning until coated. Put on broiler pan (on middle rack in oven, or at least 5 to 6 inches away from the heat source) and broil until chicken starts to brown (approximately 8-10 minutes). Brush wings with melted butter and turn. Broil for an additional 8-10 minutes, or until brown and bubbly and juices run clear. Yield: 3 servings.

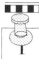

Tip: Utilize the seasoning section of your grocery store! Try Cajun seasoning, Seasoned Salt, Garlic Butter seasoning, etc. to create new and exciting variations of chicken wings. Also, don't forget the Buffalo Chicken Wings and Barbecued Chicken-Little "Legs" found in the Appetizers section of this book.

Baked Chicken

Carbs/Serving: .13g.

1 whole chicken (2-3 lbs). 1 tsp. garlic salt *(or to taste)*
1 stick butter, *melted* 1/4 tsp. lemon pepper *(or to taste)*

Rinse chicken inside and out. (Be sure to remove neck and organ package). Place chicken in a roasting pan. Brush with melted butter. Sprinkle with seasonings. Add 1/2 cup water to bottom of roasting pan, to prevent chicken from sticking. Cover with lid or foil. Bake at 350° for approximately 1 hour or until juices at inner thigh run clear when pierced with a fork. Baste with butter 2-3 times during cooking. Yield: 4 servings.

Variation 1: Omit garlic salt and lemon pepper and substitute the following:

1/2 tsp. dried marjoram, *crushed* 1/4 tsp. celery salt
1/4 tsp. dried thyme, *crushed* 1/8 tsp. pepper

Variation 2: Omit garlic salt and lemon pepper and substitute:

1/2 tsp. dried basil, *crushed* 1/2 tsp. salt
1/2 tsp. ground sage

The biggest secret to the success of <u>Baked Chicken</u> (and other roasting recipes) is using an enamel-ware roasting pan—the kind that your mother or grandmother always used to use. It will help seal in the moisture and juices and helps anything roast to perfection.

Chicken Cordon Bleu

Carbs/Serving: 1g

4 boneless, skinless chicken breasts *(thawed)*
4 slices ham
4 slices Swiss cheese
Butter and oil for frying

Place chicken breasts between two sheets of waxed paper or plastic wrap. Using a meat mallet, pound chicken breasts until very thin (about 1/4" thickness). In a large skillet, melt 2 tablespoons of butter (and 1 or 2 teaspoons of oil) at a time over medium heat. Fry chicken breasts until no longer pink in the center. Remove from skillet and let cool until able to handle. Put a slice of ham and a slice of cheese on each chicken breast, roll up jellyroll style and secure with a toothpick if needed. Bake at 350° for 15-20 minutes or until chicken is golden and cheese is melted. Yield: 4 servings.

Tip: When frying foods in butter, add a small amount of oil to help keep butter from scorching.

You can do so many things with chicken breasts—and that is why we like them so well! We buy the large "stock-up" bags of frozen boneless, skinless chicken breasts so we are able to create whatever dish strikes our fancy in a short amount of time. Along with the preceding recipe (Chicken Cordon Bleu), here is a selection of both "flat" and "rolled" chicken breast recipes that our families really enjoy!

Pan-Fried Chicken Breasts

Carbs/Serving: 0g.

4 boneless skinless chicken breasts (about 2 pounds total)
Butter and Oil for frying

In a skillet, melt 2 tablespoons of butter (and oil) at a time over medium heat. Fry chicken breasts in butter and oil, turning meat until both sides are golden brown and the inside is no longer pink. Yield: 4 servings.

(These are delicious as is—we love the butter flavor—but you can go on to create the following variations):

Cheddar-Sauced Chicken Breasts

Carbs/Serving: 2.68g.

1 recipe Pan-Fried Chicken Breasts	
Paprika	1/3 C. chicken broth
2 T. butter	1/2 C. dairy sour cream
1 C. fresh mushrooms, *sliced*	1/2 C. cheddar cheese, shredded
2 T. green onion, *sliced*	

In a saucepan, melt butter over low heat. Sauté mushrooms and green onion until vegetables are tender. Add sour cream, chicken broth, and cheddar cheese. Continue to cook gently to allow cheese to melt and become fully incorporated. Sprinkle Pan-Fried Chicken Breasts with Paprika, and spoon hot Cheddar Sauce over chicken. Yield: 4 servings.

> Tip: If the sauces that you create are too thin for your liking, then you may choose to thicken them with cornstarch. 1 tablespoon of cornstarch mixed with 1/4 cup of cold water will thicken up to 2 cups of a sauce, and add 7g. of carbs to the entire recipe. So, for example, Cheddar-Sauced Chicken Breasts (with cornstarch added), would have 4.43g instead of 2.68g—which still isn't bad for a tasty, filling dish!

Tarragon-Sauced Chicken

Carbs/Serving: 2.45 g.

1 recipe Pan-Fried Chicken Breasts
1/2 C. cold water
1/4 C. dry white wine
1 T. cornstarch
1 T. lemon juice
2 tsp. instant chicken bouillon granules
1 tsp. dried tarragon, *crushed*

In a saucepan, stir together water, wine, cornstarch, lemon juice, bouillon, and tarragon. Cook over low to medium heat until thickened and bubbly, stirring often. Spoon sauce over Pan-Fried Chicken Breasts. Yield: 4 servings.

This variation is a little fancier—which may be just right for a dinner party with friends. They'll never know how simple it was to make or that they are eating a low-carb meal!

Italian-Style Chicken Breasts
Carbs/Serving: 1.91g

1 recipe Pan-Fried Chicken Breasts
1/4 C. Contadina Pizza Sauce
12-16 pepperoni slices
1 (8oz.) pkg. mozzarella cheese, *shredded*

Place Pan-Fried Chicken Breasts in an oven-proof serving dish. Top each chicken breast with 1 tablespoon pizza sauce, 3-4 pepperoni slices, and sprinkle with cheese. Place under broiler and broil for 1-2 minutes, or until cheese is melted and golden. Yield: 4 servings. (This often helps stave off pizza cravings!)

Mushroom and Swiss Chicken Breasts
Carbs/Serving: 2.91g

1 recipe Pan-Fried Chicken Breasts
2 (4 oz.) can mushroom pieces and stems, *drained*
2 T. butter
4 slices Swiss Cheese

In a small pan, melt butter over medium heat. Sauté mushrooms in butter until golden. Place Pan-Fried Chicken Breasts in an oven-proof serving dish. Top each piece with one slice of cheese. Place under broiler and broil for 1-2 minutes, or until cheese is melted and golden. Spoon mushrooms over cheese and serve. Yield: 4 servings.

Chicken "Enchiladas"
Carbs/Serving: 2.41g

1 recipe Pan-Fried Chicken Breasts
1/2 C. prepared enchilada sauce
1 (8oz.) pkg. Cheddar Cheese, *shredded*

Place Pan-Fried Chicken Breasts in an oven-proof serving dish. Top each piece with up to 2 tablespoon of enchilada sauce, and sprinkle cheese over all. Place under broiler and broil for 1-2 minutes, or until cheese is melted and golden. If you wish, serve with cut lettuce and sour cream. Yield: 4 servings.

As you can see, Pan-Fried Chicken Breasts is just the start of some really great dinner entrees. Perhaps you can think of other variations that will be palate pleasers for your family!

Chicken Breasts Stuffed with Mozzarella

Carbs/Serving: 1.44g

4 boneless skinless chicken breasts
3 T. butter, *softened*
salt and pepper to taste
4 (1oz) slices mozzarella cheese
1-2 eggs, *beaten*
1 1/2 C. pork rind crumbs (See Tip Box, page 72)
4 T. butter, *melted*
1 T. parsley
1/8 tsp. dried sage
1/8 tsp. dried rosemary
1/8 tsp. dried thyme
1/4 C. dry white wine

Preheat oven to 350°. Place chicken between 2 sheets of wax paper. With a meat mallet, flatten to 1/4" thickness. Spread softened butter evenly over one side of each chicken breast. Sprinkle with salt and pepper. Top each with a slice of cheese. Roll up, starting with the long side; secure with toothpicks. Dip each roll in egg and dredge in crumbs. Place in an ungreased 8" square baking dish. Combine melted butter and next 4 ingredients; drizzle over chicken. Bake, uncovered, for 20 minutes. Pour wine over chicken. Bake an additional 10 minutes or until chicken is done. Yield: 4 servings.

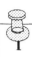

Pork Rind Crumbs for Breading and Binding
We're not sure who first discovered that pork rind crumbs can be used for breading and binding, but we sing their praises! When you need a substitute for flour, cracker crumbs, or bread crumbs, pork rinds will often fit the bill. We use them for crunchy coatings on fried meats, cheeses, and vegetables as well as a binding substance for many items from stuffed mushrooms to tuna patties. If you have never tried this wonderful "invention", then we heartily encourage you to do so. It will open up your crunchy, "batter-coated" world again with no carbohydrates!

<u>To make pork rind crumbs</u>, semi-crush the pork rinds with your hands and then place in a blender, food processor, or food chopper and continue crushing until you have fine crumbs—the finer the better. One 4oz. bag of pork rinds will produce approximately 2 cups of crumbs.
(We like to crush up several bags at a time, and keep the crumbs in an air-tight container in the refrigerator for quick breading convenience.)

Bacon-Cheddar Chicken Rolls

Carbs/Serving: .94g.

- 1 C. pork rind crumbs
- 2 tsp. snipped parsley
- 1/4 tsp. paprika
- 1/8 tsp. dried marjoram, *crushed*
- 4 boneless skinless chicken breasts
- 1/2 C. cheddar cheese, *shredded*
- 4 slices bacon, *crisp-cooked, drained, and crumbled*
- 2 eggs, *slightly beaten*
- 4 T. butter

Stir together first 4 ingredients. Set aside. Place chicken pieces, between 2 pieces of wax paper; flatten with a meat mallet to form a rectangle about 1/8" thick. Place cheddar cheese and bacon on each chicken breast. Roll up jelly-roll style and secure with a toothpick. Dip each roll in egg, and roll in seasoned pork rind crumbs. Melt butter in a large skillet over medium heat. Fry each chicken roll, turning until all sides are golden brown and done throughout. Yield: 4 servings.

Chicken Kiev

Carbs/Serving: .56g.

- 4 boneless skinless chicken breasts (about 2 pounds total)
- 1/2 of a 1/4-pound stick butter, *chilled, and cut into 4-2 1/2" long sticks*
- 2 T. chopped chives
- 2 T. chopped parsley
- 1/4 tsp. pepper
- 1/2 tsp. garlic salt
- 1 egg, beaten
- 1 C. pork rind crumbs
- 4 T. butter

Place chicken pieces, between 2 pieces of wax paper; flatten with a meat mallet to form a rectangle about 1/8" thick. Set chicken aside. In a small dish, mix together the seasonings. Roll each stick of butter in this seasoning mix. Place one of the seasoned butter sticks in the center of each chicken breast; fold over the long edges and roll up jelly-roll fashion so that the butter is completely enclosed. Secure with a toothpick. Dip each roll in beaten egg; roll in pork rind crumbs. Melt butter in a large skillet over medium heat. Fry each roll, turning until all sides are golden brown and done throughout. Yield: 4 servings.

Chicken Rolls Amandine
Carbs/Serving: 3.65g.

8 slices bacon
1 C. fresh mushrooms, *chopped*
2 T. snipped chives
1/2 C. slivered almonds
1/4 tsp. dried thyme, *crushed*
4 boneless skinless chicken breasts(about 2 pounds)
Butter and oil for frying
Plain dairy sour cream *(optional)*
Sliced almonds, toasted *(optional)*
Snipped chives *(optional)*

For filling, in large skillet fry bacon until crisp. Drain off fat, reserving 2 tablespoons drippings. Drain bacon on paper towels; crumble and set aside. Add mushrooms and 2 T. chives to reserved drippings in dish. Cook until tender. Stir in bacon, 1/2 C. almonds, and thyme. Place chicken pieces between 2 pieces of clear plastic wrap or wax paper and pound lightly with a meat mallet to form a rectangle about 1/8" thick. Remove plastic wrap or paper. Sprinkle 1 side of each chicken breast with salt and pepper. Place about 2 tablespoons of filling on the seasoned side of each chicken piece. Roll up jelly-roll style and secure with a toothpick. Melt 4 tablespoons of butter (and oil) at a time over medium heat and fry each chicken roll, turning until all sides are golden brown and done throughout. If desired, serve chicken with a dollop of sour cream (add 1 gram of carbs for each 2 T. used); sprinkle with almonds (add 1.4 gram of carbs for each additional tablespoon) and chives. Yield: 4 servings.

Crunchy Fried Chicken Breasts

Carbs/Serving: .3g.

4 boneless skinless chicken breasts
1-2 eggs *(slightly beaten)*
2 C. pork rind crumbs, *ground fine for breading*
1/2 tsp. onion or garlic salt *(or more to taste)*
Oil for frying

In a large skillet, pour oil to a depth of 1/4"-1/2". Heat oil over medium-high heat. Combine pork rind crumbs with seasoning; set aside. Rinse chicken pieces, dip in egg. Roll each chicken breast in seasoned pork rind crumbs. Fry in oil until brown on one side; then turn. Continue frying until done and juices run clear when pierced with fork, approximately 15 minutes total. Yield: 4 servings.

Chicken Nuggets

Instead of leaving the chicken breasts whole, you can slice the chicken into strips and then nugget-sized chunks before dipping in egg and breading. Fry until done and you have home-made chicken nuggets (which both you and your children will just love!)

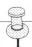

Tip: **Crunchy Fried Chicken Breasts** is a general recipe for frying many varieties of meat. Please try this with pork cutlets, pork chops, cube steak, and fish. You can also vary the seasonings with a change in pork rinds. Try the Hot and Spicy or the Barbecue flavors of pork rinds to change the flavor.

Marinades provide seasoning and tenderizing for relatively few carbohydrates. Here are just a few of the lowest carb. possibilities:

Lawry's Brand: Mesquite with Lime (1g/1T.)
　　　　　　　　Lemon Pepper (1g/1T.)
　　　　　　　　Red Wine (1g/1T.)
　　　　　　　　Sun-Dried Tomato and Basil (3g/2T)
　　　　　　　　Southwest (3g/2T.)

Golden Dipt Southwest-Style Marinade
Adolph's "For the Grill", Cracked Pepper w/lemon (2g/2 T.)

Be sure to check out the dry marinade mixes in your favorite store for flavors that we may have missed. Also, don't forget the marinade recipes in the <u>Sauces</u> section of this book!

Grilled Marinated Chicken Breasts

Carbs/Serving: 1.66-3g (Depending upon marinade chosen)

4 boneless, skinless chicken breasts, *thawed*
1/2 C. marinade (homemade, bottled or from prepared mix)

In a shallow dish, place chicken breasts, and pour marinade over all. Turn chicken until all surfaces are completely coated. Allow to marinate for 30 minutes to an hour (or according to package or bottle suggestion). Remove chicken from marinade, reserving marinade for basting. Meanwhile, prepare outdoor grill. When coals are ashed-over and medium hot, grill chicken until no longer pink in the center (approximately 15-25 minutes per side). Yield: 4 servings.

To broil: Place on broiler pan, approximately 5-6 inches from heat source, and broil for approximately 15-20 minutes per side, or until no longer pink in the center.

For either method of cooking, be sure to periodically baste chicken with reserved marinade.

Chicken Monterey

Carbs/Serving: 2g.

4 boneless skinless chicken breasts
1/2 C. Lawry's Mesquite with Lime Marinade
4 slices bacon, *crisp fried and broken in half*
4 slices Monterey Jack cheese

Prepare chicken breasts according to directions for <u>Grilled Marinated Chicken Breasts</u>. Approximately 1 minute before removing chicken from grill or broiler, place 1 slice of cheese on each chicken breast. Allow to remain on grill or under broiler until cheese is melted and bubbly. Remove from heat. Place 2 pieces of bacon on each chicken breast. Yield: 4 servings.

Chicken Amandine

Carbs/Serving: 1.41g

1/2 C. sliced almonds
1/4 C. butter
8 boneless skinless chicken breasts
1-2 eggs, *beaten*
1 1/2 C. pork rind crumbs
1/4 tsp. dried rosemary, *crushed*
1/4 tsp. salt
1/4 tsp. pepper
1/2 C. dry white wine

In a large skillet, melt butter; sauté almonds in butter over medium heat until lightly browned. Remove almonds with a slotted spoon, reserving butter in skillet. Set almonds aside. Combine crumbs, rosemary, salt and pepper. Dip chicken in egg, and roll in seasoned crumbs. Brown chicken breasts in reserved butter over medium high heat 4 minutes on each side. Stir in wine; cover, reduce heat, and simmer 15 minutes or until chicken is done. Remove chicken to a serving place, reserving juices in skillet. Set chicken aside and keep warm. Bring juices to a boil; stir in reserved almonds. Spoon almond mixture over chicken. Yield: 8 servings.

Chicken in Cream Sauce

Carbs/Serving: 3.90g

4 boneless skinless chicken breasts	1/2 C. cream
3 T. butter	1 tsp. salt
1/3 C. onion, *chopped*	1/8 tsp. pepper
1 clove garlic, *minced*	1 T. cornstarch
1/2 C. chicken broth	1/4 C. cold water
2 tsp. Worcestershire sauce	

Preheat oven to 325°. In a skillet, melt butter or heat oil; brown chicken on both sides. Transfer to a baking dish. In same skillet with drippings, combine onion, garlic, broth, cream and seasonings. Heat thoroughly, but do not boil. Pour mixture over chicken. Cover dish with foil. Bake for 45 minutes, or until chicken is no longer pink in the center. Uncover pan and bake for an additional 15 minutes. Remove chicken to a serving dish; keep warm. Blend together cornstarch and water, and add to pan sauce; cook until thickened and bubbly. Pour over chicken. Yield: 4 servings.

Sesame Chicken

Carbs/Serving: 2.03g.

4 boneless, skinless chicken breasts	Sauce
1 egg, *beaten*	2 T. butter, *melted*
1 T. water	1/2 C. chicken broth
3/4 C. Pork Rind Crumbs	1 T. soy sauce
4 T. butter	3 T. sesame seeds

In a small bowl, mix together egg and water. Dip chicken breasts in egg mixture, and then roll in crumbs to coat. In a skillet, melt butter, and pan-fry breasts until golden and crispy. Remove from skillet and place in baking dish. To make sauce, combine 2 T. melted butter, chicken broth, and soy sauce. Pour sauce over chicken breasts and sprinkle with sesame seeds. Bake at 350° for 35-40 minutes, or until chicken is completely done (no longer pink in the center). Yield: 4 servings.

Chicken Chow Mein

Carbs/Serving: 5.65g.
3 T. butter
2 T. onion, *minced*
1/2 lb. lean pork (as from chops or pork steak), *diced*
1/2 C. chicken stock
3/4 C. celery, *diced*
5 C. cooked chicken, *diced*
1 (4oz.) cans mushroom stems and pieces, *drained*
2 T. soy sauce
1/2 C. slivered blanched almonds

Melt butter in large skillet over low heat. Add onion, cook for 2 minutes. Add pork and cook until pork is browned on all sides. Drain off juices. Add chicken stock, celery, chicken and mushrooms; simmer for 10-15 minutes, until hot throughout and celery is just crisp-tender. Add soy sauce and almonds. Yield: 4 servings.

Whoever said that certain dishes *had* to be served over rice, pasta, or noodles? Our personal practice is to serve any of these "type" dishes without the designated "base". For example, Chicken Chow Mein is *always* served without rice; Stroganoff is served without noodles; (Fajitas are served without the tortillas, for that matter). This way, we can enjoy all of these wonderful low carb. recipes without the high carb. "extra baggage". Granted, sometimes a certain dish is somewhat "juicy"—so we drain off some of the juice, or serve the entree in a bowl. When you change your mind-set about your eating patterns, you will find that you can be very creative in eliminating unnecessary carbohydrates from your diet.

Garlic Chicken

Carbs/Serving: 5.48g.
1/2 C. water
2 T. soy sauce
1 T. dry white wine
1 tsp. cornstarch
4 boneless skinless chicken breasts
2 T. cooking oil
1 C. green onions, *bias-sliced into 1" pieces*
1 C. fresh mushrooms, *thinly sliced*
7 cloves garlic, *peeled and finely chopped*

For marinade, in a bowl stir together water, soy sauce, wine, and cornstarch. Rinse chicken and pat dry. Cut chicken into 1/2" pieces. Add chicken to marinade; stir to coat. Let stand at room temperature for 30 minutes. Drain chicken, reserving marinade. Preheat a wok or large skillet over high heat; add oil. (Add more oil as necessary during cooking). Stir-fry green onions, mushrooms, and garlic in hot oil for 1 to 2 minutes or until tender. Remove from wok or skillet. Add chicken to wok or skillet; stir-fry for 2 to 3 minutes or until no longer pink. Push chicken from center of wok or skillet. Stir reserved marinade; add to center of wok or skillet. Cook and stir until thickened and bubbly. Add onion mixture. Cook and stir about 1 minute or until heated through. Yield: 4 servings.

Santa Fe Chicken

Carbs/Serving: 5.6g.

4 slices bacon, *coarsely chopped*
4 boneless skinless chicken breasts, *cut into cubes*
1/2 C. onion, *chopped*
1 med. green pepper, *sliced*
1 med. sweet red pepper, *sliced*
1 tsp. ground cumin
1/2 tsp. garlic powder
1/2 tsp. chili powder
1/4 C. chopped fresh cilantro *(optional)*

Cook bacon in a large skillet over medium heat 4 minutes. Add chicken and onions; cook 6 minutes, stirring frequently. Add the next 5 ingredients and cook, uncovered, 10 minutes or until chicken is done, stirring frequently. Sprinkle with chopped fresh cilantro, if desired. Yield: 4 servings.

Herb-Marinated Chicken

Carbs/Serving: 1.13g.

2 to 2 1/2 lb. meaty chicken pieces
1/2 C. white wine
2 T. olive or cooking oil
1 T. vinegar
1/2 tsp. onion salt
2 tsp. dried basil, *crushed*
1 tsp. dried oregano or tarragon, *crushed*
2 cloves garlic, *minced*

Rinse chicken. Place chicken pieces in a large (gallon-size) plastic zipping bag. For marinade: In a bowl combine remaining ingredients. Pour over chicken pieces in the bag. Close bag and turn to coat chicken well. Marinate for 5 to 24 hours in refrigerator, turning bag occasionally. Drain chicken, reserving marinade. Place the chicken, skin side down, on the unheated rack of a broiler pan. Brush with some of the marinade. Broil 4 to 5" from heat source about 20 minutes or until lightly browned, brushing often with marinade. Turn chicken, skin side up, and broil for 5 to 15 minutes more, or until tender and no longer pink, brushing often with the marinade. Yield: 4 servings.

Royal Barbecued Chicken

Carbs/Serving: 1.26g

1 C. butter	2 tsp. dried leaf oregano
3/4 C. lemon juice	4 fryers, *halved*
2 tsp. garlic salt	3 tsp. salt
2 T. paprika	1/2 tsp. pepper

To make marinade: Melt butter in small saucepan; stir in lemon juice, garlic salt, paprika, and oregano. Set aside. Place chickens in a shallow dish; sprinkle with salt and pepper. Pour marinade over chickens; cover. Marinate for 3 to 4 hours, turning occasionally. Drain, reserving marinade. Place chicken, skin side up, on grill set 3 to 6" from charcoal briquets that have reached light gray ash stage. Brush generously with reserved marinade. Cook for 45 minutes to 1 hour and 15 minutes or until tender, turning and brushing with marinade occasionally. Leg should twist easily out of thigh joint and pieces should feel tender when probed with fork when chicken is done.
Yield: 8 servings.

Chicken Dijon

Carbs/Serving: 1.88g

2 T. butter	1/4 tsp. salt
1 (3-lb.) chicken, *quartered*	1/4 tsp. pepper
2 C. dry white wine	2 egg yolks, *beaten*
1/4 tsp. dried tarragon	2 T. sour cream
Pinch of thyme	2 T. Dijon mustard
1 bay leaf	Pinch of Cayenne pepper

In a large skillet, melt butter. Add chicken and cook until browned on all sides. Add wine and seasonings. Bring to a boil. Cover, and reduce heat to a simmer; simmer for 45 minutes or until chicken is tender. Remove chicken to heated serving dish; keep warm. Discard bay leaf. Blend sauce with egg yolks (See Tip Box, next page); add sour cream, mustard, and cayenne pepper. Heat through, stirring constantly; do not boil. Pour sauce over chicken. Yield: 4 servings.

Chicken with Lemon Sauce

Carbs/Serving: 2.06g.

2 frying chickens, *cut into pieces*
6 C. water
1 onion, *sliced*
4 celery tops, *chopped*
2 bay leaves
2 tsp. salt
1/2 tsp. peppercorns
1/4 C. butter
1 T. cornstarch
1/4 C. cold water
3 egg yolks
1/4 C. lemon juice
1/2 C. finely chopped parsley

Place chicken in a kettle or stock pot; add next 6 ingredients. Cover tightly; bring to a boil. Reduce heat; simmer for 1 hour or until chicken is tender. Place chicken on serving platter; keep warm. Strain and reserve 3 cups broth. Melt butter in saucepan and add reserved broth. Blend together cornstarch and cold water. Slowly add cornstarch mixture to broth and butter, stirring constantly. Continue cooking and stirring until thickened and bubbly. Beat egg yolks with lemon juice. (Follow tip below to keep eggs from curdling.) Add warmed egg yolk mixture to remaining sauce, stirring rapidly. Cook until mixture returns to a boil. Remove from heat; stir in parsley. Spoon half the sauce over chicken. Pour remaining sauce into a serving bowl. Yield: 8 servings.

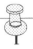

Tip: When adding egg yolks to a hot sauce, first mix a small amount of the sauce to the yolks to gently warm the eggs. Continue adding sauce until the eggs are hot, then incorporate all of the egg mixture into the sauce. This will keep the eggs from curdling.

Chicken Paprika

Carbs/Serving: 5.34g

2 (3-lb.) chickens, *cut into pieces*
2 T. cooking oil
1 C. onion, *thinly sliced*
2 T. paprika
1 1/2 C. water
Salt and pepper to taste
1 T. cornstarch
1/4 C. cold water
1 1/2 C. sour cream

Heat oil in a large skillet or Dutch oven. Brown chicken in oil. Add onion, paprika, salt and pepper, and 1 1/2 C. water; cover. Simmer for about 30 minutes. Mix cornstarch with cold water. Blend in sour cream. Add sour cream mixture to chicken, coating pieces. Simmer until sauce is heated through. Yield: 8 servings.

Roast Turkey Breast

Carbs/Serving: 0g

1 turkey breast from 3 1/2 lbs. to 7 lbs. (allow 1/2 to 3/4 lb. per serving)
1/2 C. butter, *melted*

Preheat oven to 450°. Rinse and dry the turkey breast. Place the breast on a rack in a shallow pan. Brush with melted butter. Place turkey in oven and reduce heat to 325° and roast uncovered, basting frequently, about 20 minutes per pound (or until meat thermometer registers 180° at the meat's thickest point). Yield: 7-14 servings.

Turkey Stir-Fry

Carbs/Serving: 3.25g.

4 C. leftover roast turkey, *cubed*
2 T. butter
2 (14 oz.) cans Fancy Mixed Chinese Vegetables (by LaChoy), *drained*
2 (4 oz.) cans mushroom stems and pieces, *drained*
1 T. soy sauce (or to taste)

In a skillet, melt butter and sauté turkey until golden. Stir in drained vegetables and mushrooms. Add soy sauce. Continue cooking until vegetables are hot. Yield: 4 servings.

Beef

> Ground beef is such a versatile food-stuff that you could probably (if you chose to) serve some version of it every day of the week without boring your family. Additions of seasonings and other low-carb ingredients will turn the ordinary, sometimes "dull" hamburger into a tasty treat that your family will really enjoy.

Hamburgers

Carbs/Serving: 0g.
2 lb. ground beef, *Shaped into 1/2"- 3/4" thick patties*
Salt (or onion salt) and pepper to taste

To pan-fry: Preheat a large skillet slowly, over medium heat. (Meat should sizzle, not hiss sharply, when added to pan.) Fry burgers, uncovered for 3 or 4 minutes. Turn. Sprinkle fried side with salt and pepper. Continue frying for another 3-4 minutes, or until juices run clear when the burger is pressed with a spatula.

To broil: Place burgers on a broiler pan, 4 inches from source of heat. Broil for 6 minutes on one side, turn, and broil an additional 4 minutes on the other side. Salt and pepper to taste.

To grill: Before shaping beef into patties, add 1 beaten egg to meat, then shape burgers. (This will help the meat to hold together better on the grill.) When coals have reached the light-gray ashed-over stage, place burgers on grill rack. Grill approximately 6 minutes to a side, or until burgers are gray in the center, and the juices run clear. Add salt, pepper, and/or barbecue sauce (see Sauces section), if desired. (Grilled burgers costs approximately .15g/serving.) Yield: 4 servings.

Variations of the traditional hamburger:

Cheeseburger

Carbs/Serving: 0-1g (Depending upon cheese chosen)

1 recipe Hamburgers, prepared as you desire
1 (1oz.) slice cheese for each burger

Prepare burgers according to direction for Hamburgers. Approximately 1 minute before burgers are done, add one slice of cheese to each, and continue cooking until burgers are done and cheese is melted. Yield: 4 servings.

Note: You can really create a variety of cheeseburgers just by varying your choice of cheese, rather than staying with the traditional American cheese. Try Provolone, Pepper-Jack, Swiss, Muenster, Cheddar, Colby, Colby-Jack, etc.

Ranchburgers

Carbs/Serving: 3.64g

2 lbs. ground beef
1 pkg. dry Ranch Dressing Mix

Mix ground beef and dressing mix. Shape into patties. Cook burgers according to the directions for Hamburgers. Yield: 4 servings.

Pizzaburgers

Carbs/Serving: 1.91g

1 recipe Hamburgers
1/4 C. Contadina Pizza Sauce
Pepperoni slices
1 (1oz.) slice mozzarella cheese per burger

Prepare hamburgers according to directions for Hamburgers. 1 minute before burgers are done, spread 1/2 to 1 tablespoon pizza sauce on each burger. Place 3-4 pepperoni slices and 1 slice of mozzarella cheese atop each burger. Continue cooking until burgers are done and cheese is melted. Yield: 4 servings.

Taco burgers
Carbs/Serving: 1.46g
1 recipe Hamburgers
1 T. taco sauce for each burger
1-2 T. shredded cheddar cheese for each burger

Prepare hamburgers according to directions for Hamburgers. 1 minute before burgers are done, sprinkle cheese on each burger. Continue cooking until burgers are done and cheese is melted. Spread taco sauce over each burger. Serve with shredded lettuce and sour cream, if desired. Yield: 4 servings.

Mushroom/Swiss burgers
Carbs/Serving: 1g.
1 recipe Hamburgers
1 (1oz.) slice Swiss cheese per burger
1 (4oz.) can mushroom stems and pieces, *drained*
2 T. butter

In a small pan, melt butter over medium heat. Sauté mushrooms until golden. Remove from heat and set aside. Prepare hamburgers according to directions for Hamburgers. 1 minute before burgers are done place 1 slice cheese on each burger. Continue cooking until burgers are done and cheese is melted. Spoon mushroom and butter sauce over each burger.
Yield: 4 servings.

Salisbury Steak
Carbs/Serving: 2.24g
1 Recipe Hamburgers
1 C. Mushroom Gravy Sauce (pg. 146)

Preheat oven to 350°. Prepare burgers according to directions for (Pan-Fried) Hamburgers. When burgers are well browned on both sides, remove burgers from skillet and place in a baking dish. Pour mushroom gravy sauce over the burgers. Bake for 20-30 minutes, or until burgers are done (gray in the center).
Yield: 4 servings.

Meatloaf
Carbs/Serving: .80g

2 lb. ground beef	1/4 tsp. pepper
1 egg, *beaten*	2 tsp. Worcestershire sauce
1/4 C. pork rind crumbs	1/2 C. green pepper, *chopped*
1 1/2 tsp. onion salt	6 slices bacon

Preheat oven to 350°. In a mixing bowl, combine all ingredients (except bacon slices) until well mixed. Pat out ground beef mixture into a 9x13" baking pan. Top with bacon slices. Bake for 45 minutes to 1 hour, until meat loaf is a light gray in the center and juices run clear. Pour off fat and water that has been rendered. Allow to set for 10 minutes. Transfer meatloaf to a serving platter just before serving. Yield: 6 servings.

Stroganoff
Carbs/Serving: 4.91g

2 T. butter	1 tsp. onion salt
2 (4oz.) cans sliced mushrooms, *drained*	1/4 tsp. pepper
	1/2 C. water
2 lb. ground beef	1 tsp. beef bouillon granules
	1 C. sour cream

In a large skillet, melt butter. Sauté mushrooms until golden. Remove mushrooms and butter from skillet and set aside. In the same skillet, brown ground beef over medium heat until meat is gray. Drain off excess fat. Add next 4 ingredients, stirring well. Add sour cream and mushrooms to the meat mixture, and continue cooking just until the mixture is hot throughout. Yield: 4 servings. (Remember, we feel that there is no need to serve this with noodles, despite traditional convention. It is delicious and hearty on its own!)

Variation: Instead of ground beef, you may use 2 lb. stew meat (or round steak, sliced into 1/2" thick strips—although the meat is somewhat tougher). After sautéing the mushrooms and removing them from the skillet, add an additional 2 T. butter to the skillet. Slowly, sauté beef over medium heat until done. Continue recipe as above.

Border Chili

Carbs/Serving: 4.74g.

2 lb. ground beef
1/4 C. chopped onion
1 tsp. garlic powder
1/4 tsp. cumin
1/4 tsp. oregano
1 tsp. salt
1/4 tsp. red pepper, *optional*
1/4 C. chili powder
2 C. hot water
1 T. cornstarch
1/4 C. cold water

In a skillet, sauté beef and onion over medium heat until beef is no longer pink. Add the next 7 ingredients. Simmer until beef is tender. Mix cornstarch with cold water; add to chili mixture gradually stirring until thickened. Simmer for 15 minutes longer. Serve with shredded cheddar cheese and sour cream, if desired. But....skip the crackers! Yield: 6 servings.

Southwest Casserole

Carbs/Serving: 4.97g

2 lb. ground beef
1 (8oz.) can tomato sauce
1 tsp. garlic powder
1 tsp. onion salt
Dash pepper
1/4 tsp. oregano
2 1/2 tsp. chili powder
1/2 C. heavy cream
1 T. cornstarch
1/4 C. cold water
1/4 C. grated Parmesan cheese

Preheat 350°. In a skillet, brown beef over medium heat; drain excess fat. Stir in next 6 ingredients; mix well. Reduce heat. Stir in cream. Mix cornstarch with cold water, and add to beef mixture gradually, stirring well. Transfer mixture to a 9x13" (or slightly smaller) baking dish. Sprinkle casserole with Parmesan cheese. Bake for 20-25 minutes. Serve with shredded cheddar cheese and sour cream, if desired. Yield: 6 servings.

Sloppy Joes

Carbs/Serving: 3.79g

2 1/2 lb. ground beef
1/2 C. celery, *chopped*
1/2 C. green bell pepper, *chopped*
1 3/4 C. Sweet and Smoky Barbecue Sauce (pg. 144)
1/2 C. water, *optional*
Salt and pepper to taste

In a large skillet, brown ground beef over medium heat. Drain well. Add celery, and green pepper. Continue cooking until vegetables are crisp-tender. Add barbecue sauce and water, if desired to meat mixture. Reduce heat to low, cover, and simmer for about 15 minutes or until mixture is somewhat thickened. (Spoon onto plates, not sandwich buns.) Yield: 6 servings.

Gravy-Sauced Meatballs

Carbs/Serving: 3.68g

2 lbs. ground beef
2 eggs, beaten
1/2 C. pork rind crumbs
1 tsp. onion salt
3 T. chopped parsley
1/4 tsp. paprika
1 tsp. lemon juice
1 tsp. Worcestershire sauce

3 T. butter
2 C. beef stock
1 T. cornstarch
1/4 C. cold water

In a large mixing bowl combine the first 8 ingredients, mixing until well combined. Shape into 1" meatballs. In a skillet, melt butter over medium heat and brown meatballs on all sides. Add beef stock to skillet, reduce heat, cover, and simmer meat for 15 minutes. Remove meatballs from stock and set aside. Combine cornstarch and cold water. Add cornstarch mixture to hot stock stirring continually. Cook until thickened. Add meatballs back to gravy, stirring to coat. Continue to cook until meatballs are thoroughly heated. Yield: 4 servings.

Swedish Meatballs

Carbs/Serving: 4.51g

Following the above recipe, omit the Worcestershire sauce, and add instead:
- 1/4 tsp. nutmeg
- 1/8 tsp. allspice

Continue recipe as instructed. To the pan gravy add:
- 2 T. to 1/4 C. sour cream
- 1 tsp. dillweed, *optional*

Remove to a serving dish. Sprinkle with a light garnish of paprika, if desired. Yield: 4 servings.

Reuben Burgers

Carbs/Serving: 1.3g.
- 2 (12oz.) cans corned beef
- 2 eggs, *beaten*
- 2/3 C. pork rind crumbs
- Oil for frying
- 1 (1oz.) slice Swiss cheese per burger
- Sauerkraut
- Reuben Sauce (Sauces Section, pg. 148)

In a medium sized mixing bowl, break up corned beef into small pieces. Add beaten eggs and pork rind crumbs. Mix together, stirring until well-blended. Shape mixture into patties. In a large skillet, fry patties in oil over medium heat until bottom side is golden; turn patty. Top each patty with 1 slice of Swiss cheese and continue frying until cheese is melted and patty is done. Remove to a serving plate. If desired, top each patty with 1-2 tablespoons of sauerkraut and serve with Reuben Sauce. Yield: 4 servings.

Pot Roast

Carbs/Serving: 2.41g

1 (2 1/2 to 3lb.) beef chuck pot roast
2 T. cooking oil
3/4 C. water or dry cooking wine
1 T. Worcestershire sauce
1 tsp. instant beef bouillon granules
1 tsp. dried basil, *crushed*
1 tsp. onion powder
1/2 tsp. celery salt
1 T. cornstarch
1/4 C. cold water

In a Dutch oven, brown roast on all sides in hot oil. Drain fat. In a small mixing bowl, combine the next 6 ingredients. Pour sauce over roast. Bring to boiling; reduce heat. Cover and simmer 1 hour 45 minutes to 2 hours, or until meat is tender—adding additional water if necessary. Remove meat from pan. For gravy, measure pan juices; skim fat. If necessary, add water to equal 1 3/4 cups. Return juices to pan. Combine cornstarch and cold water. Stir into pan juices. Cook and stir until thickened and bubbly. Cook and stir 1 minute more. Season to taste. Makes 10 servings.

To make in the oven: Preheat oven to 325°. Brown meat as above in a large skillet. Combine next 6 ingredients. Pour over roast. Bake, covered in a roasting pan for 1 hour 45 minutes to 2 hours or until tender. Prepare gravy as above, using a saucepan.

To make using a slow-cooker: Brown meat as above in a large skillet. Place meat in 3 1/2 to 4 quart electric slow cooker, cutting roast to fit if necessary. Combine next 6 ingredients. Pour over roast. Cover; cook on low-heat setting for 10 to 12 hours. Prepare gravy as above, using a saucepan.

Barbecued Beef Pot Roast

Carbs/Serving: 5.81g

1 (2 1/2 to 3 lb.) beef chuck pot roast
2 T. butter
1 C. onion, *sliced*
2 cloves garlic, *minced*
3/4 C. bottled barbecue sauce*
1 4oz. can sliced mushrooms, *drained*
1 T. dry mustard
1 tsp. chili powder
1/2 C. water

In a Dutch oven, brown meat on all sides in butter. Remove meat. Add onions and garlic. Cook until tender but not brown. Stir in barbecue sauce, mushrooms, dry mustard, chili powder, and water. Add meat. Bring to boiling; reduce heat. cover; simmer for 1 1/2 to 2 hours or until meat is tender, basting meat occasionally. Remove meat; boil pan juices gently for 3 to 5 minutes or to desired consistency, stirring often.
Yield: 10 servings..
*If possible, try to use Hunt's Light Barbecue Sauce (6g/2T.). **Or**, use one of the barbecue sauce recipes listed in the <u>Sauces</u> section of this book to lower the carb count to 2.95g or 3.29g.
To make in the oven: Preheat oven to 325°. Brown meat as above in a large skillet. Remove meat to an oven roasting pan. Sauté onions and garlic in skillet. Stir in remaining ingredients. Bring sauce to boiling; pour over roast. Bake, covered in a roasting pan for 1 hour 45 minutes to 2 hours or until tender. Continue preparing sauce as above, using a saucepan.
To make using a slow-cooker: Brown meat as above in a large skillet. Place meat in 3 1/2 to 4 quart electric slow cooker, cutting roast to fit if necessary. Sauté onions and garlic in skillet. Stir in remaining ingredients. Bring sauce to boiling; pour over roast. Cover; cook on low-heat setting for 10 to 12 hours. Continue preparing sauce as above, using a saucepan.

Herbed Rump Roast

Carbs/Serving: 1.97-2.36g.

1 (3 to 4lb.) boneless beef round rump roast
2 T. cooking oil
1 C. onion, *chopped*
1 tsp. instant beef bouillon granules
1 tsp. dried marjoram, *crushed*
1 tsp. dried thyme, *crushed*
1 bay leaf
1 clove garlic, *halved*
1/2 C. water
1/4 tsp. pepper
1 T. cornstarch
1/4 C. cold water
1 T. snipped parsley

In a Dutch oven, brown roast on all sides in hot oil. Drain fat. Combine the next 8 ingredients and add to Dutch oven. Bring to boiling; reduce heat. Cover; simmer 1 3/4 to 2 1/4 hours or until meat is tender. Remove meat from pan. Discard bay leaf and garlic. For gravy, measure pan juices; skim fat. If necessary, add water to equal 1 3/4 cups. Combine cornstarch, 1/4 C. cold water, and parsley. Stir into juices. Return to pan. Cook and stir until thickened and bubbly. Cook and stir for 1 minute more. Season to taste. If desired, sprinkle with additional snipped parsley. Yield: 10-12 servings.

To make in the oven: Preheat oven to 350°. Brown meat as above in a large skillet. Transfer meat to an oven roasting pan. Combine the next 8 ingredients and pour over roast. Bake, covered for 1 3/4 to 2 1/4 hours or until meat is tender. Continue as above, preparing gravy in a saucepan.

To make in a slow-cooker: Brown roast as above in a large skillet. Transfer meat to a 3 1/2-4 quart electric slow-cooker. Combine the next 8 ingredients and pour over meat. Cover; cook on low-heat setting for 10-12 hours. Prepare gravy as above, using a saucepan.

Italian Beef

Carbs/Serving: .40g-.49g

1 (3 1/2-4lb.) boneless rolled rump roast or boneless arm roast
2 T. cooking oil
2 tsp. basil
1 tsp. onion salt
1 tsp. red pepper, *crushed*
1/2 tsp. garlic powder
1 tsp. oregano
2 C. water

In a Dutch oven, brown roast on all sides in hot oil. Drain fat. Sprinkle seasonings over meat. Add water to Dutch oven. Cover; simmer 1 3/4 to 2 1/4 hours or until meat is tender. Yield: 10-12 servings.

To make in the oven: Preheat oven to 325°. Brown meat as above in a large skillet. Transfer meat to an oven roasting pan. Sprinkle seasonings over meat. Add water to roasting pan. Bake, covered for 1 3/4 to 2 1/4 hours or until meat is tender.

To make in a slow-cooker: Brown roast as above in a large skillet. Transfer meat to a 3 1/2-4 quart electric slow-cooker. Sprinkle seasonings over meat. Add water to slow-cooker. Cover; cook on low-heat setting for 10-12 hours.

Marinated Steaks

Carbs/Serving: 1.66-3g (depending upon marinade chosen)
4 (1 1/2" to 2" thick) steaks (sirloin, T-bone, strip, or porterhouse)
1 C. marinade (bottled, made from mix, or recipe from <u>Sauces</u> section)

Rinse steaks. In a large shallow pan, place steaks. Pierce both sides of steaks in several places with a long-tined cooking fork. Pour marinade over meat. Cover and refrigerate for 1 to 4 hours, (or according to directions on bottle or package, if using commercial marinades). Be sure to turn meat periodically.

<u>To grill:</u> Prepare grill, and when coals have reached a light-gray ash stage, place steaks on rack. Cover grill, and cook meat until desired doneness, turning periodically to ensure even grilling. Baste often with reserved marinade or melted butter.

<u>To broil:</u> Preheat broiler. Place steaks on broiler rack approximately 3-4 inches from the heat source. Allow to broil 8-10 minutes per side, depending on steak thickness and desired doneness. Baste with reserved marinade or melted butter.
Yield: 4 servings.

Country-Fried Steak

Carbs/Serving: 1.7g (If you skip the gravy, the carbs are almost nil)
6 cube steaks, *mechanically tenderized from your butcher*
1 egg, *beaten*
2 C. pork rind crumbs
Salt, onion powder, and pepper to taste
3 T. oil
2 C. beef stock (can be made from beef bouillon granules)
1 T. cornstarch
1/4 C. cold water

Rinse steaks; pat dry. Dip each steak in beaten egg and then roll in the pork rind crumbs. Heat oil in a large skillet over medium heat. Fry each steak in the hot oil until golden on both sides, and ash-gray in the center. Sprinkle with seasonings as desired. Remove meat from skillet and drain briefly on paper towels. In the skillet, loosen coating and drippings left from frying. Add beef stock to the drippings. In a small bowl, combine cornstarch with cold water. Slowly add to hot stock, stirring continually. Cook until thickened. Season with salt and pepper as desired. Serve hot steaks with the pan gravy on the side.
Yield: 6 servings.

Fajitas

Carbs/Serving: 5.03g

1 clove garlic, *minced*
1 1/2 tsp. chili powder
1-2 pkts. sweetener
1 tsp. oregano
1/4 tsp. red pepper
1 tsp. cumin
1/4 C. oil
1/4 C. water
2 tsp. salt
2 lbs. round steak, *sliced into 1/2" thick strips*
1 C. onion, *sliced into strips*
1 green bell pepper, *sliced into strips*
1 red bell pepper, *sliced into strips*
Oil for frying

Mix together first 9 ingredients. Place meat in a shallow pan or a heavy plastic zipping bag. Pour marinade over meat, stirring or turning bag to thoroughly coat meat. Marinate meat in this mixture for 1-2 hours in refrigerator. Preheat a large skillet and add 2-4 tablespoons oil. Drain meat of excess marinade. When oil is hot, fry meat until almost done. Add onions and peppers, and continue cooking until meat is done, and vegetables are crisp-tender. Serve with shredded cheddar cheese and sour cream. But, leave the tortillas at the store! Yield: 6 servings.

Variation: Use chicken breasts sliced into strips, or shelled, deveined shrimp in place of (or along with) beef.

Swiss Steak

Carbs/Serving: 4.88g

- 2 lb. round steak
- 1 tsp. garlic powder
- 2 T. oil
- 1/2 C. onion, *chopped*
- 1/2 C. green bell pepper, *chopped*
- 1/2 C. celery, *chopped*
- 1 C. hot water
- 1 tsp. beef bouillon granules
- 1 (8oz.) can tomato sauce
- Salt and pepper to taste

Preheat oven to 300°. Sprinkle round steak with garlic powder. With a meat mallet, pound the steak on both sides to help tenderize. Cut into serving-size pieces. In a large skillet, heat oil over medium heat and sear steak on both sides until brown. Remove steak to a baking dish. Top steak with vegetables. Mix together hot water, beef bouillon granules, and tomato sauce. Pour over steak. Cover baking dish and bake for 1 1/2 to 2 hours. Yield: 6 servings.

Steak and Green Peppers

Carbs/Serving: 2.96g

- 2 lb. round steak
- 1/4 C. Kikkoman soy sauce
- 1 C. hot water
- 1 tsp. beef bouillon granules
- 1 tsp. garlic powder
- 1/2 tsp. ginger
- 3 T. oil
- 1/2 C. water
- 2 C. green bell pepper, *sliced into strips*

Slice steak into 1/2" thick strips. Combine the next 5 ingredients in a medium bowl. Add meat to this marinade, stirring until thoroughly coated. Cover, and marinate in the refrigerator for 2 to 12 hours, stirring meat periodically. Drain meat, discarding marinade. Dry meat slightly on paper towels. In a large skillet, heat oil over medium heat. Stir-fry meat in oil until browned on all sides. Add 1/2 cup water to pan, cover, and simmer for 20-30 minutes, adding more water as necessary. Stir in green pepper strips and continue to cook, uncovered, for an additional 5-10 minutes, or until meat is done and peppers are crisp-tender. Yield: 6 servings.

Beef Goulash

Carbs/Serving: 5.95g

2 lb. stewing beef, *cut into 1" cubes*
1/4 C. butter or oil
1 1/2 C. onion, *chopped*
1 C. beef stock *(you may need more throughout the cooking)*
1 green bell pepper, *diced*
1 tsp. salt
1 tsp. paprika
1 T. cornstarch
1/4 C. cold water

In a large skillet or heavy pot, melt butter (or heat oil) over medium heat. Brown meat on all sides in the hot butter or oil. Add onion and sauté until golden. Add remaining ingredients. Reduce heat. Cover, and simmer the meat for 1 1/2 hours. When meat and vegetables are done and tender, remove from pot. Set aside and keep warm. Measure juices remaining in pot. Add water or stock until the juices measure 2 cups. Return stock to pan. Combine cornstarch and cold water. Slowly add cornstarch mixture to hot stock, stirring continually. Continue cooking until gravy is thickened. Pour gravy over meat and vegetables, or serve on the side, as you desire.
Yield: 6 servings.

> The next recipe is a little fancier and more time-consuming. But, when you need a break from standard "Sunday Dinner" fare, or something more special for the holidays, Steak Roll With Dressing may be what you're looking for. Our families feel very special when we take the time to make this tasty dish!

Steak Roll with Dressing

Carbs/Serving: 3.61g

2 to 3 lb. flank or round steak
1 tsp. salt
1/8 tsp. paprika
1/4 tsp. dry mustard
1 tsp. Worcestershire sauce
1/4 C. butter
2 T. onion, *chopped*
1 C. pork rind crumbs
1/4 tsp. salt
Dash paprika
2 T. chopped parsley
3 T. chopped celery
1 egg, beaten
3 T. oil
1 C. beef stock (you may make this with bouillon granules, if desired)
1 C. dry red wine
1/4 tsp. salt
1 T. cornstarch
1/4 C. cold water

Preheat oven to 300°. Sprinkle steak with first 4 ingredients. With a meat mallet, pound steak on both sides to tenderize. In a small pan, melt butter over medium heat. Add next 7 ingredients and sauté in the butter to make a dressing. Spread this dressing over the steak, roll loosely—jelly-roll fashion, and tie it with butcher string. In a large skillet, heat oil over medium heat. Sear the rolled steak on all sides in the hot oil. Place in a baking dish. In the skillet add the beef stock, wine, and salt. Combine the cornstarch with the cold water, and gradually add this mixture to the stock and wine. Cook until thickened. Pour this mixture over the steak roll. Bake, covered, about 1 1/2 hours. Season as desired. Yield: 6 servings.

Pork

Pork Roast

Carbs/Serving: 1.31g

1 (3 to 5 lb.) pork loin or shoulder roast	1 tsp. onion salt
2 T. cooking oil	1 tsp. garlic powder
1 C. water or dry white wine	1 T. cornstarch
1 tsp. dried rosemary or thyme, *crushed*	1/4 C. cold water

In a Dutch oven, brown roast on all sides in hot oil. Drain fat. In a small mixing bowl, combine the next 4 ingredients. Pour sauce over roast. Bring to boiling; reduce heat. Cover and simmer 2 to 3 hours, or until internal temperature reaches at least $140°$, the center of the roast is white or a light gray, and the juices run clear. You may need to add additional water as necessary to keep roast from drying out during cooking. Remove meat from pan. Allow to rest for 10-15 minutes before slicing and serving. Serve with pan gravy, if desired.

For gravy, measure pan juices; skim fat. If necessary, add water to equal 1 3/4 cups. Return juices to pan. Combine cornstarch and cold water. Stir into pan juices. Cook and stir until thickened and bubbly. Cook and stir 1 minute more. Season to taste. Makes 8 to 10 servings.

To make in the oven: Preheat oven to $325°$. Brown meat as above in a large skillet. Combine next 4 ingredients. Pour over roast. Bake, covered in a roasting pan for 2-3 hours or until done as described above. Prepare gravy as above, using a saucepan.

To make using a slow-cooker: Brown meat as above in a large skillet. Place meat in 3 1/2 to 4 quart electric slow cooker, cutting roast to fit if necessary. Combine next 4 ingredients. Pour over roast. Cover; cook on low-heat setting for 10 to 12 hours, or until done as described above. Prepare gravy as above, using a saucepan.

Barbecued Pork Roast

Carbs/Serving: 5.41g

1 (2 1/2 to 3 lb.) pork loin or shoulder roast	2 cloves garlic, *minced*
	3/4 C. bottled barbecue sauce*
2 T. butter	1 T. dry mustard
1 C. water	1 tsp. chili powder
1 C. onion, *chopped*	1/2 C. water

In a Dutch oven, brown meat on all sides in butter over medium heat. Add water. Reduce heat. Cover and simmer for 2 to 3 hours or until meat is done as described for Pork Roast. (Add more water to pan as necessary.) Remove meat. Allow meat to stand for 15 minutes before slicing or shredding. Meanwhile, to pan juices add onions and garlic. Simmer until tender. Stir in remaining ingredients. Add sliced or shredded meat. Simmer sauce and meat gently uncovered for 3 to 5 minutes or to desired consistency, stirring often. Yield: 10 servings.

*To lower carbs to 2.55-2.89g/serving, use one of the barbecue sauce recipes listed on pages 144 or 145.

To make in the oven: Preheat oven to 325°. Brown meat as above in a large skillet. Remove meat to an oven roasting pan. Add water to pan. Bake, covered for 2 to 3 hours or until done as described for Pork Roast. Allow roast to rest as described above. In skillet, simmer onions and garlic in pan juices removed from roasting pan. Stir in remaining ingredients; add shredded roast. Continue preparing as above.

To make using a slow-cooker: Brown meat as above in a large skillet. Place meat in 3 1/2 to 4 quart electric slow cooker, cutting roast to fit if necessary. Add water to slow cooker. Cover; cook on low-heat setting for 10 to 12 hours, or until done as described for Pork Roast. Remove meat from slow cooker; allow to rest for 15 minutes before slicing or shredding. In a skillet, simmer onions and garlic in pan juices. Stir in remaining ingredients. Continue preparing as above.

Pork Roast Stir-Fry

Carbs/Serving: 3.25g.

4 C. leftover pork roast, *cubed*
2 T. butter
2 (14 oz.) cans Fancy Mixed Chinese Vegetables (by LaChoy), *drained*
2 (4oz.) cans mushroom stems and pieces, *drained*
1 T. soy sauce (or to taste)

In a skillet, melt butter and sauté pork until golden. Stir in drained vegetables and mushrooms. Add soy sauce. Continue cooking until vegetables are hot. Yield: 4 servings.

Sautéed Pork Chops

Carbs/Serving: .5g.

4 pork chops, 1/2"-1" thick
3 T. cooking oil or butter
Salt, pepper, garlic powder, and/or lemon pepper to taste

Rinse meat and pat dry. In a large skillet, heat butter or oil over medium heat. Sear pork chops on both sides. Reduce heat and continue to cook chops slowly until done. Season with salt, pepper, and/or garlic powder to taste. Yield: 4 servings.

Baked Pork Chops

Carbs/Serving: .5g

4 pork chops, 1" or more thick
3 T. cooking oil or butter
1/2 C. water

Salt, pepper, garlic powder, and/or lemon-pepper to taste

Preheat oven to 350°. Rinse meat and pat dry. In a large skillet, sear chops as described for Sautéed Pork Chops. Remove chops to a baking dish and add water. Bake, covered for about 1 hour. During the last 30 minutes of baking, sprinkle chops with desired seasonings. Yield: 4 servings.

Broiled or Grilled Pork Chops

Carbs/Serving: 1.66-3g (Depending upon marinade chosen)

4 pork chops, 1/2"-1" thick
1/2 C. marinade (bottled, prepared mix, or recipe from Sauces Section)

Rinse chops and pat dry. In a shallow dish, place chops; pour marinade over all, turning to coat each chop thoroughly. Marinate for 1 to 2 hours, or as per commercial marinade instructions. Remove chops from marinade, reserving excess for basting. Place chops on a broiler rack approximately 5-6 inches from the heat source. Broil, for approximately 15-20 minutes per side, until light gray in the center. Baste periodically with reserved marinade or melted butter.

To grill: Prepare outdoor grill. When coals are ashed-over, and medium hot, grill chops until light gray in the center (approximately 15-25 minutes per side). As with broiling, baste periodically with reserved marinade or melted butter.

Breaded Fried Pork Chops

Carbs/Serving: .32g

4 pork chops, 1/2" thick   1/2 tsp. garlic salt
1 egg, *beaten*   1/4 tsp. black pepper
2 C. pork rind crumbs   3 T. butter

Rinse meat and pat dry. In a large skillet, melt butter over medium heat. Dip chops in beaten egg, and roll in crumbs seasoned with garlic salt and pepper. Fry chops in butter until golden on both sides. Reduce heat and continue to cook uncovered for about 20 minutes longer, or until tender. Yield: 4 servings.

To bake instead of fry: Preheat oven to 350°. Place breaded chops in a baking dish or on a broiler rack. Bake, uncovered for 1 hour, turning after 30 minutes. If chops appear to be drying out, you may top each with 1/2 T. butter.

Breaded Pork Cutlets (with Pan Gravy)

Carbs/Serving: 2.15g (If you skip the gravy, the carbs are almost nil)
6 pork cutlets
1-2 eggs, *beaten*
2 C. pork rind crumbs
Salt, onion powder, and pepper to taste
3 T. oil
1 C. chicken stock (can be made from chicken bouillon granules)
1/2 C. heavy whipping cream
1 T. cornstarch
1/4 C. cold water

Rinse cutlets, and pat dry. Dip each cutlet in beaten egg and then roll in the pork rind crumbs. Heat oil in a large skillet over medium heat. Fry each cutlet in the hot oil until golden on both sides. Reduce heat and continue to cook slowly until meat is ash-gray in the center. Sprinkle with seasonings as desired. Remove meat from skillet and drain briefly on paper towels. In the skillet, loosen coating and drippings left from frying. Reduce heat to low. Add chicken stock and cream to the drippings. In a small bowl, combine cornstarch with cold water. Slowly add to hot stock, stirring continually. Cook until thickened, but do not boil. Season with salt and pepper as desired. Serve cutlets with the pan gravy on the side. Yield: 6 servings.

Barbecued Pork Steak

Carbs/Serving: 2.48 to 3.6g, (depending on barbecue sauce chosen)
4 pork steaks
Salt and pepper to taste
1 C. barbecue sauce (from <u>Sauces</u> section of this book, pages 144 or 145)

<u>To Broil:</u> Place pork steak on broiler rack 5-6" from heat source. Broil for approximately 15-20 minutes per side, or until center of steaks is light gray. As one side finishes cooking, sprinkle steaks with salt and pepper. Brush on barbecue sauce. Turn steaks and broil remaining side. Repeat seasoning and brushing on sauce for the remaining side. Allow to broil one more minute to "brown" barbecue sauce slightly. Turn steaks to "brown" sauce for one more minute. Yield: 4 servings.

To grill: Prepare outdoor grill. When coals are at the light-gray ashed over stage, place steaks on rack of grill. Grill steaks for approximately 15-20 minutes per side, or until center is light gray. As with broiling, do not season or add sauce until turning the meat away from the source of heat. Grill the remaining side. Season and sauce as before. Yield: 4 servings.

Country-Style Ribs

Carbs/Serving: 4g.

4 lb. spareribs or country-style ribs, cut into 2" pieces
1/2 C. barbecue sauce, (See page 144 or 145, or use Hunt's Light)
1/2 C. butter, *melted*

Place ribs in a large stock pot and cover with water. Bring to a boil; reduce heat and continue to simmer for 1 to 1 1/2 hours or until meat is gray at its most central point. Drain ribs. Combine barbecue sauce and melted butter. Set aside until needed for basting.

To broil: Place parboiled ribs on broiler rack approximately 5-6" from heat source. Baste with barbecue/butter sauce, and broil until glazed and crispy.

To grill: Prepare grill. When coals are ashed-over, place parboiled ribs on grill rack. Baste with barbecue/butter sauce, and grill until glazed and crispy. Yield: 6 servings.

Pork Chow Mein

Carbs/Serving: 5.22g

2 lb. lean pork steak
1/2 C. onion, *chopped*
1 C. celery, *sliced*
3 T. soy sauce
1 C. water
1 tsp. beef bouillon granules

1 T. cornstarch
1 (4oz.) can sliced mushrooms, *drained (reserve 1/4 C. liquid)*
2 (14 oz.) cans La Choy Fancy Mixed Chinese Vegetables, *drained*

Trim excess fat from meat. Cut steak diagonally into very thin strips. Lightly grease large skillet with excess fat; brown meat on both sides. Stir in onion, celery, soy sauce, and broth made from water and bouillon granules. Cover; simmer 30 minutes. Blend cornstarch and reserved mushroom liquid; gradually stir into meat mixture. Add mushrooms, and Chinese vegetables. Continue cooking and stirring until vegetables are hot, and sauce is thickened. Yield: 6 servings. (No rice, please!)

Mediterranean Pork

Carbs/Serving: 5.10g

2 lb. lean, boneless pork steak, cut into 3/4" cubes
1 T. cooking oil
1 tsp. onion powder
2 cloves garlic, *minced*
1 tsp. instant chicken bouillon granules
1 C. water
1 tsp. dried thyme, *crushed*
1/8 tsp. pepper
1 (4oz.) can sliced mushrooms, *drained*
1/4 C. sliced pitted ripe olives *(optional)*
2 T. snipped parsley
2 tsp. cornstarch
1/4 C. cold water

In a large skillet, heat oil over medium heat. Brown pork in hot oil. Add the next 6 ingredients. Bring to boiling; reduce heat. Cover; simmer 45 minutes or until tender. Skim fat, if necessary. Stir in mushrooms, olives (if desired), and parsley. Combine cornstarch with cold water; stir into pork mixture gradually. Cook and stir until thickened and bubbly. Cook and stir for 1 minute more. Yield: 4 servings.

Baked Ham

Carbs/Serving: 1.16g

1 (5-7 lb.) fully cooked ham (make sure label states 0g. carbs/serving)
1/2 C. butter, *melted*
2 tsp. prepared mustard
1/2 tsp. ground cloves
Sweetener to equal 1/2 cup sugar

Preheat oven to 325°. To heat the ham, place in a roasting pan. Cover and bake until the internal temperature reaches 140° (allow approximately 18 to 20 minutes per pound). Meanwhile, prepare basting sauce by combining melted butter, mustard, cloves, and sweetener. During the final 30 minutes of baking, remove cover, score top of ham with diagonal (diamond shaped) gashes, and brush all over with basting sauce. Baste several times during this final baking period. Remove ham to a serving platter. Yield: 10-14 servings.

Ham Steak
Carbs/Serving: .3g
1 (2 lb.) ham steak, about 1" thick
2 T. butter
Onion powder, if desired, to taste

In a large skillet, melt butter over medium heat. Brown ham steak on one side; turn. Sprinkle browned side lightly with onion powder, if desired. When both sides are browned and steak is hot, remove to a serving platter. Yield: 4 servings.

To broil: Place ham steak on a broiler rack, approximately 3 inches from heat source. Broil 8 to 12 minutes per side. Before turning broiled side away from heat source, brush with melted butter and sprinkle with onion powder. Turn, and continue broiling. 1 minute before second side is finished, brush with butter and sprinkle with onion powder, if desired. Yield: 4 servings.

Grilled Italian Sausages
Carbs/Serving: 4.95g
8 Italian sausage links
1 medium green bell pepper, sliced into strips
1 C. onion, sliced into strips
2 T. oil

Prepare grill. When coals are ashed-over, place sausage links on grill rack. Grill, turning often to ensure even cooking, until sausages are gray in the center and juices run clear. Remove links from the grill. While links are gilling, heat oil in a skillet over medium heat. Sauté pepper and onion until vegetables are crisp-tender. Serve grilled sausages with pepper-onion mixture. Yield: 4 servings.

Stuffed Bratwurst

Carbs/Serving: 5g

8 bratwurst links
1 C. sauerkraut
8 slices bacon
1/4 C. barbecue sauce (Try recipes on pg. 144-145 to lower carb count)
1/4 C. butter, melted

If bratwursts are not fully cooked, then fill a saucepan with enough water to just cover the links, and boil them for approximately 10-12 minutes, or until done. Remove from water, and allow to cool. When cool enough to handle, split bratwursts lengthwise to form a slit or pocket on one side. Stuff this pocket with 1-2 T. of sauerkraut. Wrap each bratwurst with one slice of bacon and secure with toothpicks. In a small bowl, combine barbecue sauce and butter. Set aside until ready to baste bratwursts. Yield: 4 servings.

To broil: Place stuffed bratwursts on broiler rack about 4-5" from the heat source. Broil, turning bratwursts until bacon is cooked and crispy on all sides. Baste with barbecue/butter sauce.

To grill: Prepare grill. When coals are ashed-over, place stuffed bratwursts on grill rack. Grill, turning bratwursts until bacon is cooked and crispy on all sides. As with broiling, baste with barbecue/butter sauce.

Variation: You may also choose to substitute polish sausage (Kielbasa) links for the bratwursts. Read labels carefully, though. Some cheaper brands are full of sugar and fillers, and are therefore rather high in carbs. But, some brands (i.e., Boar's Head and Jones Dairy Farm Dinner) have 0-1g/serving.

Polish Sausage and Sauerkraut

Carbs/Serving: 3.5g

1 lb. Kielbasa polish sausage, *cut into 1 inch pieces*
2 T. butter
1 (14.4 oz.) can sauerkraut, *drained*

In a large skillet, melt butter over medium heat. Lightly sauté sausage in butter until heated and golden. Add sauerkraut and continue heating until hot throughout. Yield: 4 servings.

Italian Sausage "Burgers"

Carbs/Serving: 4.51g

1 lb. bulk Italian sausage
1/4 C. Contadina Pizza Sauce
1 (4oz.) can mushroom stems and pieces, *drained*
4 (1oz.) slices mozzarella cheese

Preheat oven to 375°. Shape sausage into 4 1/2-thick patties. In a skillet, cook sausage patties until no pink remains in the center. Drain fat. Place patties in a small oven-proof baking dish. In a small mixing bowl, combine pizza sauce and mushrooms. Spoon sauce mixture over patties. Top each patty with 1 slice of cheese. Bake until cheese is melted and patties are hot. Yield: 4 servings.

Side Pork

Carbs/Serving: .15g

1 lb. side pork, *sliced thick*
1 egg, *beaten*
2 C. pork rind crumbs
Oil for frying

In a large skillet, heat oil over medium heat. Dip each slice of pork in beaten egg and roll in crumbs. Fry in hot oil, turning until both sides are golden and crispy. Yield: 4 servings.

Fish

"Blackened" Fish Fillets

Carbs/Serving: 1-1.5g, (depending upon amount of seasoning used)
4-6 fish fillets (roughy, whiting, perch, etc.), *thawed*
1/2 C. butter, *melted*
Blackened Seasoning, *to taste*
Salt, to taste

Preheat oven to 350°. Rinse thawed fish. Pat dry with paper towels. Place fillets in a shallow baking dish. Brush both sides generously with melted butter, and sprinkle with seasonings. Bake approximately 15-20 minutes; turn fillets and bake an additional 15-20 minutes (depending upon size and thickness of the fillets). Fish will flake with a fork when done, and flesh will be an opaque white color. To achieve a crusty brown appearance, place baked fillets under the broiler for 3-5 minutes per side, or to desired doneness. Yield: 4 servings.

Variation: Omit the Blackened Seasoning and substitute Lemon-Pepper Seasoning, or dillweed and chives.

Baked Fish with Mushrooms

Carbs/Serving: 1.9g
1 lb. (1/2"-3/4" thick) fish fillets, *thawed*
1 C. fresh mushrooms, *sliced*
1/2 C. green onion, *sliced*
1/4 tsp. dried tarragon, *crushed*
2 T. butter
Paprika

Preheat oven to 450°. Rinse fish and pat dry. Grease 9"x13" baking dish with butter, oil, or cooking spray. Arrange fillets in the baking dish, turning under thin edges. Sprinkle with salt. In a small pan, melt butter. Cook mushrooms, onion, and tarragon in butter until tender. Spoon over fish; sprinkle with paprika. Bake, covered, for 6 to 10 minutes, or until fish flakes easily with a fork. Yield: 4 servings.

Cajun Catfish Fillets

Carbs/Serving: .3g.
10-12 catfish fillets
2 eggs, *beaten*
4 C. pork rind crumbs
2 tsp. Cajun seasoning (Durkee's or Tone's)
Salt and pepper to taste
Oil for frying

Heat oil in a deep fat fryer to recommended depth, or in a large, heavy saucepan to a depth of 4 inches. Heat oil to 370°. Rinse fillets. Pat dry with paper towels. Dip fillets in egg, then roll in crumbs seasoned with Cajun seasoning, salt, and pepper. Deep fry in oil for 5-8 minutes, or until golden brown, and tender-white in the center. Drain on paper towels. Serve with Homemade Tartar Sauce (pg.148)
Yield: 4-6 servings.

Variation: Omit Cajun seasoning, and substitute 1 tsp. onion salt and 1/2 tsp. garlic powder. Also, you may use fish fillets other than catfish, (such as whiting, orange roughy, perch, etc.).

Tip: When deep-frying meat, fish, or vegetables, one indicator that the food is done cooking will be that it floats to the surface.

Southwestern Grilled Fish

Carbs/Serving: 3g.
4-6 fish fillets
1 C. "Golden Dipt" Southwest-style marinade

Rinse fish fillets and pat dry. Place fillets in a shallow dish, and pour marinade over all, turning until fish is thoroughly coated and covered. Marinate for 30-45 minutes in the refrigerator. Remove fish from marinade. Place fillets on a *large* square of heavy aluminum foil that has been lightly oiled. Fold sides of foil to create a pocket, tightly crimping all edges*. Prepare grill. When coals are ashed-over, place foil packet on grill rack. Grill about 20 minutes; turn package, and grill an additional 20 minutes. 5 minutes before fish is done, open foil packet to give the fish some additional "smoky" flavor. Yield: 4 servings.

*Tip: Crimp edges tightly, but do not wrap the fish tightly. If you leave a little room in the pocket of the aluminum foil, it will give the fish room to steam, and ensure better cooking.

Fish Fillets Amandine

Carbs/Serving: 2.9g

4-6 fish fillets
1 egg, *beaten*
2 C. pork rind crumbs
4 T. butter
1/2 C. slivered almonds

Rinse thawed fish, and pat dry. Melt 2 T. butter in a large skillet over medium heat. Sauté fillets in hot butter, turning once. Continue cooking until fish is crispy, golden and flakes easily with a fork, about 3 to 5 minutes per side depending on size and thickness of fillets. Remove fish to a hot platter. In skillet, melt remaining 2 T. butter. Add almonds and brown lightly. Pour almonds and butter over fish fillets. Yield: 4 servings.

Tuna Patties

Carbs/Serving: 1.11g

4 (6oz.) cans tuna, *drained*
1 C. pork rind crumbs
1 egg, *beaten*
1 T. mayonnaise
1/2 tsp. onion salt
1 T. dill relish, *optional*
1 tsp. horseradish, *optional*
1 (8oz.) pkg. cheddar cheese, *shredded (optional)*
3 T. oil (add more oil as needed)

In a mixing bowl combine all ingredients, except cheese and oil. Shape tuna mixture into small (3-4" diameter) patties. In a skillet, heat oil over medium heat. When oil is hot, fry tuna patties for 2-3 minutes per side, or until golden, crispy, and hot throughout. Remove to a baking dish. Top patties with shredded cheese, if desired. Place under broiler for 1-2 minutes or until cheese is melted and bubbly. Serve with Tartar Sauce (pg. 148). Yield: 4 servings.

Fried Popcorn Shrimp

Carbs/Serving: .55g

2 lb. raw popcorn shrimp, *peeled and deveined*
2 eggs, *beaten*
4 C. pork rind crumbs
1/2 tsp. garlic powder
Salt and pepper to taste
Oil for frying

Heat oil in a deep fat fryer to recommended depth, or in a large heavy saucepan to a depth of 4 inches. Heat to approximately 370°. Rinse thawed shrimp in a strainer. Allow to drain on paper towels. In a large plastic zipping bag, combine pork rind crumbs, garlic powder, salt and pepper. Place beaten egg in a medium bowl; add shrimp and toss to coat all pieces. Using a slotted spoon, transfer shrimp to plastic bag. Seal, and shake to thoroughly coat all shrimp pieces. Again, using a slotted spoon, remove shrimp from bag. Shake off excess breading and deep fry in hot oil until golden and crispy.
Yield: 4 servings.

Shrimp in Garlic Butter

Carbs/Serving: 1.7g

2 lb. shrimp, *peeled and deveined*
4 T. butter
4-5 cloves garlic, *minced*
3 T. snipped parsley
2 T. dry sherry, or white cooking wine

Thaw shrimp, if frozen. Rinse, and drain on paper towels. In a large skillet, heat butter over medium-high heat. Add shrimp and garlic. Cook, stirring frequently, for 1 to 3 minutes or until shrimp turns pink. (Do not overcook, as shrimp will become tough.) Stir in parsley and sherry or wine. Yield: 4 servings.

Variation: You may substitute scallops for the shrimp. Cook scallops in butter for 3-5 minutes or until the scallops turn opaque. Continue recipe as above. Yield: 4 servings.

Eggs

Eggs are a vital staple to any low-carbohydrate eating plan. They are versatile, tasty, filling, and add so much dimension to your diet. However, they can also become tedious and boring if you get stuck in a rut of eating them cooked only 1 or 2 ways. So, we encourage you to try a new recipe once in a while. You may find new dishes that your family will proclaim as "That's a keeper, Mom".

> Apology in advance: We opted to *not* fill this section with basic cooking instructions for eggs. If you are a novice cook, and are not sure about the method to fry, hard-boil, or poach an egg, then we recommend that you refer to a general cooking text to give you those instructions. We felt that you would prefer to have spent your money on tasty and interesting recipes instead.

Deviled Eggs

Carbs/Serving: .75g

6 hard-boiled eggs, *shelled*
1/4 C. mayonnaise
1 tsp. prepared mustard
1 T. dill relish, *optional*
1 pkt. sweetener, *optional*
Paprika

Halve eggs lengthwise; remove yolks. Place yolks in a bowl; mash with a fork. Add remaining ingredients; mix well until smooth. Season with salt and pepper, if desired. Stuff egg white halves with yolk mixture. Garnish with a sprinkle of paprika, if desired. Yield: 6 servings.

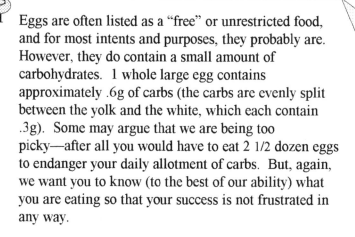

Eggs are often listed as a "free" or unrestricted food, and for most intents and purposes, they probably are. However, they do contain a small amount of carbohydrates. 1 whole large egg contains approximately .6g of carbs (the carbs are evenly split between the yolk and the white, which each contain .3g). Some may argue that we are being too picky—after all you would have to eat 2 1/2 dozen eggs to endanger your daily allotment of carbs. But, again, we want you to know (to the best of our ability) what you are eating so that your success is not frustrated in any way.

Scrambled eggs aren't just for breakfast anymore! Try some of these savory versions; add bacon, sausage, or ham and serve "breakfast" for dinner!

Cheese and Onion Scrambled Eggs
Carbs/Serving: 2.15g

8 eggs
1/3 C. heavy cream
1/2 C. cheddar, or mozzarella,
    or Swiss cheese, *shredded*
1 tsp. onion salt
Dash pepper
2 T. butter

In a bowl, beat together all ingredients, except butter. In a large skillet, melt butter over medium heat; pour in egg mixture. Cook, without stirring, until mixture begins to set on the bottom and around the edge. Using a large spoon or spatula, lift and fold partially cooked eggs so that uncooked portion flows underneath. Continue cooking over medium heat for 2 to 3 minutes or until eggs are cooked throughout but are still glossy and moist. Remove from heat immediately. Yield: 4 servings.

Variations:

Mushroom Scrambled Eggs
Carbs/Serving: 3.04g

Follow the ingredients and instructions for Cheese-Onion Scrambled Eggs, except omit: cheese. Substitute instead:

1 (4oz.) can sliced mushrooms, *drained*
1 T. snipped parsley
1/2 tsp. dry mustard
1/4 tsp. Worcestershire sauce

Yield: 4 servings.

Western (or Denver) Scrambled Eggs
Carbs/Serving: 3.33g

Follow the ingredients and instructions for Cheese-Onion Scrambled Eggs, except omit: onion salt. Substitute instead:

1 (4oz.) can sliced mushrooms, *drained*
1/2 C. fully cooked ham, *diced*
1/4 C. green bell pepper, *chopped*
1 tsp. garlic salt
1/8 tsp. pepper

Yield: 4 servings.

Italian Herbed Scrambled Eggs

Carbs/Serving: 1.5g

Follow the ingredients and instructions for <u>Cheese-Onion Scrambled Egg</u>, except omit: onion salt and cheese. Substitute instead:

1/4 tsp. salt
1 tsp. Italian seasoning blend
2-3 T. grated Parmesan cheese

Yield: 4 servings

Dinner Omelets

Carbs/Serving: 1.2g.

2 eggs   1/8 tsp. salt
1 T. water   1 T. butter

In a bowl, combine eggs, water, salt, and dash pepper. Using a fork, beat until combined but not frothy. In an 8 or 10" skillet with flared sides, heat butter until a drop of water sizzles. Lift and tilt pan to coat the sides. Add egg mixture to skillet; cook over medium heat. As eggs set, run a spatula around the edge of the skillet, lifting eggs and letting uncooked portion flow underneath. When eggs are set but still shiny, remove from the heat. Top with filling, if desired. Fold omelet in half. Transfer to a warm plate (or, if making several for dinner, transfer to a baking dish and keep covered in an oven warmed to 300°.

Yield: 1 serving.

Filling Suggestions for Dinner Omelets:

Mushroom filling:

Carbs/Serving: 1.07g
For each omelet, sauté in butter:
1/3 C. sliced fresh mushrooms, per omelet

Spoon across center of omelet. Fold sides over and remove from pan as described above.

Cheese Filling:

Carbs/Serving: .91g
For each omelet, use:
1/4 C. Cheddar, Swiss, Monterey Jack, or American cheese, *shredded*

Simply sprinkle cheese across center of omelet. Fold sides over. Remove from pan as described above. When all omelets are completed, if desired, top omelets with additional cheese and toast briefly under broiler until cheese is melted and bubbly.

Denver Filling:

Carbs/Serving: 1.6g.
For each omelet, sauté in butter:
2 T. green bell pepper, chopped
2 T. fully cooked ham, minced
2 T. green onion, chopped

Spoon across center of omelet. Fold sides over. Remove from pan as described above.

Crustless Quiche

Carbs/Serving: 4.05g.

4 eggs, *beaten*
1 1/2 C. heavy whipping cream
1/4 C. green onion, *sliced*
1/4 tsp. salt
1/8 tsp. pepper
3/4 C. cooked chicken, crabmeat, or ham, *chopped*
1 1/2 C. Swiss, cheddar, or Monterey Jack cheese, *shredded*

Preheat oven to 325°. Meanwhile, in a bowl stir all ingredients and mix well. Pour egg mixture into a greased 9" pie pan. Place pie pan into a large baking dish and pour hot water into the dish around the pie pan to a depth of 1". Bake quiche in oven for 35 to 40 minutes or until a knife inserted near the center comes out clean. Remove from oven. Let stand 10 minutes. Yield: 4 servings.

Variation: To make **Quiche Lorraine**, substitute 8 slices of crisp-cooked and crumbled bacon for the 3/4 C. meat, and use 1 1/2 cups shredded Swiss cheese. Follow instructions for Crustless Quiche. Yield: 4 servings.

For a simple and very low-carb supper or luncheon, serve Crustless Quiche or Quiche Lorraine with a simple lettuce salad (use Theresa's Vinegar-Mustard Dressing over the cut lettuce—the "tang" is just right with the quiche). Your table (and plate) may look somewhat bare, but your tummies and appetites will be totally satisfied!

Chiles Rellenos Casserole

Carbs/Serving: 4.54g

1 lb. ground beef
1 lb. ground pork, or Italian sausage
1 tsp. onion salt
1 1/2 tsp. garlic powder
1/2 tsp. chili powder
4 (4oz.) cans chopped green chilies, *drained*
2 C. cheddar cheese, *shredded*
8 eggs, *beaten*
1 tsp. hot sauce
1 1/4 C. heavy whipping cream

Preheat oven to 350°. In a large skillet, brown ground beef and pork over medium heat until done. Drain fat. Season browned meat with onion salt, garlic powder, and chili powder. In a greased 9"x13" baking dish, layer ingredients in this order: 2 cans green chilies, 1 C. cheddar cheese, browned meat, 2 cans green chilies, and remaining 1 C. cheese. In a mixing bowl, whip together until well mixed the eggs, hot sauce and cream. Pour over casserole layers. Bake for 45 minutes, or until knife inserted near center comes out clean. Remove from oven. Allow to set for 10 minutes. Serve with salsa or taco sauce and sour cream, if desired. Yield: 9 servings.

Once again, this is another recipe that is so completely satisfying that it could stand on its own as a complete meal. If desired, serve some cut lettuce along with the salsa/taco sauce and sour cream garnishes. You won't leave the table dissatisfied!

Egg-Sausage Stir-Fry

Carbs/Serving: 3.98g
1 lb. bulk pork sausage
8-10 eggs
1 C. frozen pepper stir-fry mix (red, green, yellow bell peppers)
Pinch garlic salt
Salt and pepper to taste

Brown sausage in a large skillet over medium heat. Drain excess fat, leaving about 2 T. in pan with sausage. Add peppers and stir-fry for about 3 minutes, or until peppers are heated. Add garlic salt, salt, and pepper to beaten eggs; pour egg mixture over sausage and peppers. Cook until eggs are scrambled, about 3 minutes more. Top with shredded cheddar cheese, if desired. Yield: 4 servings.

Note: If you are unable to find a frozen pepper stir-fry blend, you may substitute the following chopped vegetables: 1/2 C. green bell pepper, 1/2 C. red bell pepper, and 1/4 C. onion.

Variation: You may choose to substitute ham or bacon for the sausage. If using ham, use butter to sauté the vegetables. If using bacon, fry crisp and drain on paper towels. Reserve bacon drippings to sauté vegetables, and add crumbled, fried bacon after eggs are cooked.

Eggs Benedict

Carbs/Serving: 1.05g
4 poached eggs
8 slices Canadian bacon
Hollandaise sauce (pg. 147)

Warm Canadian bacon slices in a microwave or lightly brown in a buttered skillet. Place 2 slices of bacon on a serving plate. Top with one poached egg. Spoon Hollandaise sauce over egg and bacon. Yield: 4 servings.

Eggs in Ham Cakes

Carbs/Serving: .79g
1 C. cooked ham, *ground*
1 egg
1 T. water
1/8 tsp. paprika or pepper
4 eggs

Preheat oven to 325°. In a mixing bowl, mix together first 4 ingredients. Press 1/4 of this ham mixture into each of 4 greased muffin tins. Leave a large hollow in each one. Drop one egg into each hollow. Bake the cakes until the eggs are firm, about 10 minutes. Remove to a serving plate. Yield: 4 servings.

Variation:

Eggs in Bacon Rings

Carbs/Serving: .6g
Follow the instructions for Eggs in Ham Cakes, with the following exceptions: omit first 4 ingredients. Substitute instead 4 slices bacon that have been partially cooked. Line the sides of each greased muffin tin with one slice of bacon. Drop in each tin, if desired, 1/4 tsp. hot sauce. Drop one egg into each muffin tin. Pour over each egg 1 tsp. melted butter. Bake as directed above. Yield: 4 servings

Vegetables

Vegetables are a necessary component of our eating regimen. They provide (among other things) vitamins, minerals, and fiber. During the weight-loss phase of your eating plan, you may feel that your vegetable choices are somewhat limited, since vegetables are also a prime source for carbohydrates. If the bad news is that your choices are limited, then the good news is that your choices are healthier than the corn, beans, and potato side dishes of your former eating lifestyle. With a bit of an open mind (we never dared to try asparagus before low-carb eating!) and a need to expand your menus, you may find that there are new vegetables or new recipes destined to become family favorites—or, at the very least (by your children) well-tolerated additions to your repetoire!

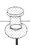

We didn't include any higher-carbohydrate vegetable recipes in this volume, as we have found that even small deviations to include a taste of corn, peas, beans, and potatoes were often enough to slow or stop our weight-loss progress. However, when you reach the maintenance phase of this lifestyle, you will be able to include some of these (and others) on a limited, strictly monitored basis. If you really begin to miss a favorite vegetable, consult your chosen program for suggestions to help you through your cravings.

Classic Green Beans

Carbs/serving: 4.0g

2 (14.5oz.) cans cut green beans, *drained*
1/2 tsp. onion salt
4 slices bacon
2 T. butter
Salt and pepper to taste

In a large pan, fry bacon until crisp; drain, reserving 4 tablespoons drippings. When cool, crumble bacon and set aside. To the reserved bacon drippings, add butter. Add beans, onion powder, and seasonings to taste. Continue sautéing until beans are well-cooked, having a glazed appearance. Add bacon to beans. Salt and pepper to taste. Makes 7 (1/2-cup) servings.

Note: You can also use frozen beans, but you need to prepare them in the microwave or on the stove according to the package directions before adding to the bacon drippings and butter.

Variation: Eliminate bacon and bacon drippings. Sauté beans in butter; add 1 pound cooked ham cubes to beans and heat through.

Green Beans in Herbed Butter

Carbs/serving: 4.49g

2 (14.5oz.) cans cut green beans, *drained*
1/4 C. butter
1 tsp. onion salt
1 clove garlic, *minced*
1/4 C. celery, *minced*
1/4 tsp. rosemary
1/4 tsp. dried basil
1T. chopped parsley

Melt butter in saucepan; add onion salt, garlic, and celery. Sauté for 5 minutes. Add remaining seasonings and beans. Simmer, covered, for 10 minutes, tossing well to coat beans with sauce. Yield: 7 (1/2 cup) servings.

Spanish-Style Green Beans

Carbs/serving: 4.49g

2 (14.5oz.) cans cut, or French-style green beans, *drained*
3 T. vegetable or olive oil
1 tsp. onion powder
1 clove of garlic, *pressed*
1/4 lb. ham, *chopped*
1/4 lb. bacon, *chopped*
1/4 C. dry white wine or water
Dash of nutmeg
Salt to taste
Pepper to taste

Heat oil in a large skillet; add onion powder, garlic, ham, and bacon. Cook until ham and bacon are done; add wine, nutmeg, salt and pepper. Add beans and small amount of water if necessary. Cover; simmer until heated through.
Yield: 7 servings.

Green Beans Amandine

Carbs/serving: 4.79g

2 (14.5oz.) cans cut or French-style green beans, *drained*
1/4 C. sliced or slivered almonds
2 T. butter
2 tsp. lemon juice

In a large skillet, cook and stir almonds in butter over medium heat until golden. With a slotted spoon, remove almonds from pan; set aside. Add beans and lemon juice to skillet (Add more butter, if necessary). Cook, stirring occasionally until beans are heated through. Stir sautéed almonds into beans.
Yield: 7 servings.

Herb-Buttered Mushrooms

Carbs/serving: 4.36g

4 C. fresh mushrooms, *sliced*
1/4 C. green onion, *chopped*
2 cloves garlic, *minced*
3 T. butter
1 tsp. dried basil, *crushed*
1/4 tsp. lemon-pepper seasoning (or, black pepper)

In a large skillet, sauté mushrooms, onions, and garlic in butter over medium-high heat until mushrooms are tender, stirring occasionally. Add basil, and lemon-pepper seasoning or pepper. Cook for 2 to 3 minutes or until heated through.
Yield: 4 servings.

Sautéed Mushrooms

Carbs/serving: 3.45g

4 C. fresh mushrooms, *sliced*
2 T. butter
1 T. oil
1 clove garlic, *peeled*

In a large skillet, melt butter and add oil; heat over medium-high heat. Add the mushrooms, stirring gently to coat with butter and oil. Drop in the garlic clove. Continue to cook, uncovered, stirring gently or simply shaking the pan for 3 to 4 minutes. Remove garlic clove. Yield: 4 servings.

Quick tip: Pan-fry canned mushroom slices in butter when you don't have time to prepare fresh mushrooms. It's a step-down, but still tasty.

Zucchini in Dill Sauce

Carbs/serving: 5.41g

4 C. zucchini, *julienned*
1/4 C. green onion, *finely chopped*
2 T. water
1 T. butter
1/2 tsp. dried dillweed
1 tsp. instant chicken bouillon granules
1/3 C. sour cream

Cut zucchini into 2"x1/4" julienned strips. In a large saucepan, combine zucchini, onion, water, butter, dillweed, and bouillon granules. Bring to boiling; reduce heat. Cover and simmer 3 to 5 minutes or until zucchini is almost tender, stirring once. Do not drain. Remove from heat. Stir sour cream into zucchini mixture. Cook and stir until bubbly. Cook and stir 1 minute more. Yield: 4 servings.

Stir-fried Squash

Carbs/serving: 5.22g

3 C. zucchini, *sliced into 1/4" thick round slices*
3 C. summer squash, *sliced into 1/4" thick round slices*
1 tsp. onion powder
1/2 tsp. garlic powder
salt and pepper
2 T. butter

In a large skillet, melt butter over medium heat. Add summer squash, zucchini, onion and garlic powders, salt, and pepper to taste. Continue cooking until vegetables are crisp-tender. Season again, if necessary. Makes 6 servings.

Variation: Add 3/4 tsp. oregano. Before serving, sprinkle with grated Parmesan cheese.

Zucchini Patties

Carbs/serving: 4.19g

- 2 med. size zucchini squash, *coarsely grated*
- 3 eggs, *beaten*
- 2/3 C. pork rind crumbs
- 1/2 tsp. garlic powder
- 1 tsp. onion power
- Salt and pepper to taste
- Butter (and oil) for frying

In a colander, place grated zucchini. Sprinkle lightly with salt to help draw out excess moisture. Place a small plate on top of zucchini, and weight down with a heavy can. Allow to drain for 30 minutes to an hour. After zucchini has drained, combine zucchini, eggs, pork rind crumbs, and seasonings in a mixing bowl until thoroughly mixed. Melt butter and oil in a large skillet. When hot, drop large spoonsful of the zucchini mixture into the butter and fry as you would pancakes. When the zucchini is set and brown on one side, turn and fry the other side. Remove to warmed serving platter. Yield: 4 servings.

"Batter"-Fried Vegetables

Carbs/serving: 4.39g-okra; 2.49g-zucchini; 2.19g-mushrooms

- 4 C. finely crushed pork rinds
- 1 tsp. onion powder
- 1/2 tsp. garlic powder
- 2 eggs, *well beaten*
- 4 C. sliced vegetables (thinly sliced okra, zucchini, or mushrooms)
- Oil for frying

Pour oil in a deep fat fryer according to manufacturer instructions; or in a large, heavy pan to a depth of 2 inches. Preheat to 400° (high). Combine pork rind crumbs, onion powder, and garlic powder until well mixed. Place on a plate or in a shallow bowl. In a small bowl, place well beaten eggs. Dip sliced vegetables, one slice at a time, into egg. Roll slices in crumbs until thoroughly coated. Fry in hot oil until golden brown, approximately 1 minute per side. Remove from oil with a slotted spoon and drain on paper towels. Yield: 8 servings.

Sesame Asparagus

Carbs/serving: 3.77g

3/4 lb. asparagus spears or (one) 10oz. pkg. frozen cut asparagus
1 T. butter
1 T. sesame seed
1 C. fresh mushrooms, *sliced*
1 tsp. lemon juice
1/4 tsp. sesame oil (optional)

Snap off and discard woody bases from fresh asparagus. If desired, scrape off scales. Cut into 1" pieces. Cook, covered, in a small amount of boiling water for 6 to 8 minutes or until crisp-tender. (Or, cook frozen asparagus according to package directions). Drain; remove from pan. In the same pan melt butter; add sesame seed. Cook and stir 2 to 3 minutes or until toasted. Add mushrooms; cook and stir until tender. Add lemon juice and, if desired, sesame oil. Add asparagus; toss to coat. Heat through. Yield: 4 servings.

Variations:

Asparagus Amandine

Carbs/serving: 3.43g

1/4 C. slivered blanched almonds
1/4 C. butter
1/4 tsp. salt
2 tsp. lemon juice
3/4 lb. asparagus spears or (one) 10oz. pkg. frozen cut asparagus

Sauté almonds in butter until golden, stirring occasionally; remove from heat. Add salt and lemon juice. Prepare and cook asparagus as directed in Sesame Asparagus. Place cooked asparagus in serving dish. Pour almond mixture over asparagus. Let stand for several minutes before serving. Yield: 4 servings.

Asparagus in Cheese Sauce
Carbs/serving: 4.16g
3/4 lb. asparagus spears or (one) 10oz. pkg. frozen cut asparagus
2 T. butter
1 pint heavy whipping cream
1/2 C. grated Cheddar cheese

In small saucepan, melt butter over low heat. Add cream and continue heating gently over *low* heat. When hot, add cheese. Continue stirring until cheese is melted and incorporated into cream. Keep cheese sauce warm and occasionally stir as you prepare the asparagus. Prepare and cook asparagus according to directions for <u>Sesame Asparagus.</u> Place in warmed serving dish. Pour cheese sauce over asparagus and serve immediately. Yield: 4 servings.

Note: The cheese sauce is a thin light sauce, but it will thicken slightly if allowed to cook longer. The key is a low flame and a bit of patience.

Winning Vegetables
Carbs/serving: 4.35g
3 C. broccoli florets
3/4 C. carrots, diced
1 C. red bell pepper, diced
2 C. small button mushrooms, washed and patted dry
5 T. butter
Salt and pepper to taste

Blanch broccoli and carrots in boiling salted water until about half-cooked. Drain well and allow to steam dry in a colander. Melt butter in a skillet and add vegetables. Quickly sauté until almost tender. Season with salt and pepper and serve immediately. Yield: 8 servings.

Note: For best flavor, vegetables should remain a little crunchy.

Golden Broccoli Bake

Carbs/serving: 4.68g

1 1/2 lbs. broccoli, cut up (6 cups), *or* one (16oz) pkg. frozen cut broccoli
1/2 C. heavy cream
1/4 C. shredded mild cheddar (or colby-jack) cheese
1 egg, beaten
1 (4oz.) can sliced mushrooms, *drained*
1 T. mayonnaise
1 T. chopped pimiento

Preheat oven to 350°. Cook fresh broccoli, covered, in a small amount of boiling water for 9 to 11 minutes or until crisp-tender. (Or, cook frozen broccoli according to package directions). Drain. Transfer to a buttered 1 1/2-quart casserole. Add mushrooms. In a small mixing bowl, combine cream, cheese, egg, mayonnaise, and pimiento. Stir into broccoli and mushrooms. Bake 30-45 minutes or until hot throughout. Yield: 8 servings.

Broccoli-Carrot Stir-Fry

Carbs/serving: 5.51g

1 T. orange peel, *grated*
1 T. dry sherry
1/4 C. chicken stock
1 tsp. cornstarch
1 T. cooking oil
1/2 tsp. ginger
1/2 C. carrots, *thinly bias-sliced*
2 1/2 C. broccoli florets
2 T. chopped walnuts

For sauce, in a bowl stir together first 6 ingredients. Set aside. Preheat a wok or large skillet over high heat. Add cooking oil. (Add more oil as necessary during cooking.) Stir-fry carrot for 1 minute. Add broccoli and stir-fry for 3 to 4 minutes or until crisp-tender. Push vegetables from the center of the wok or skillet. Stir in sauce; add to center of wok. Cook and stir until thickened and bubbly. Cook and stir for 1 minute more. Stir in vegetables and walnuts to coat. Serve immediately. Yield: 4 servings.

Chinese Broccoli

Carbs/serving: 4.83g

8 C. broccoli florets
2 T. grated onion
2 T. oil
2 T. lemon juice
2 T. Kikkoman soy sauce
Freshly ground pepper to taste

Blanch broccoli 1 minute in boiling, salted water; drain and cool. Set broccoli aside. Sauté onion in oil until onion is tender. Stir in lemon juice, soy sauce, and pepper; add broccoli and stir-fry 2 to 3 minutes or until hot throughout. Yield: 8 servings.

Cauliflower in Cheese Sauce

Carbs/serving: 5.29g

3 C. cauliflower florets
1 T. butter
1 T. cornstarch
1/4 C. cold water
1/2 C. cream
1/2 C. mild cheddar, or colby-jack cheese, *shredded*
1 (4oz.) can sliced mushrooms, *drained*

In a saucepan, cook cauliflower, covered, in a small amount of boiling water for 8 to 10 minutes or until crisp-tender. Drain; remove from pan. In the same pan, melt butter over medium heat. Add cream. In a small bowl, combine cornstarch and cold water. Stir slowly into cream and butter. Cook and stir until bubbly and thickened. Stir in cheese until melted. Add cauliflower and mushrooms; heat through. Yield: 6 servings.

Cauliflower with Almond Butter

Carbs/serving: 4.38g

4 C. cauliflower florets
Salt
1/4 C. slivered almonds
3 T. butter

Cook cauliflower in boiling salted water for 10 minutes or until tender; drain. Sauté almonds in butter until lightly browned. Place cauliflower in serving dish; pour butter and almonds over top. Yield: 6 servings.

Fried Cauliflower with Cheese Sauce

Carbs/Serving: 5.45g

4 C. cauliflower, *separated into 1" pieces*
1 tsp. salt
Cooking oil
2 eggs, *beaten*
2 C. pork rind crumbs
1/4 C. butter
2/3 C. chicken broth
1/2 C. heavy cream
1 T. cornstarch
1/4 C. cold water
1/4 C. grated Parmesan cheese

Separate cauliflower into florets. Simmer, covered, in salted water for 20 minutes or until tender. Drain and cool. Heat cooking oil in deep fryer to 400°. Dip each piece of cauliflower into eggs, then into crumbs. Fry until brown and crisp on outside. Melt butter in saucepan over low heat; add broth and cream. In a small bowl, combine cornstarch and cold water; slowly stir into cream mixture. Cook, stirring constantly until thick; fold in cheese; cover. Remove from heat. Allow cheese to melt. Stir; pour over hot cauliflower. Yield: 6 servings.

California Casserole
Carbs/serving: 5.12g

1 (16oz.) pkg. frozen California blend vegetables
1/2 C. cream
1/2 C. water
1 tsp. chicken bouillon granules
1 egg, *beaten*
1 (4 oz.) can mushrooms, *drained*
1 (8oz.) pkg. Cheddar cheese, *shredded*
Salt and pepper to taste
Butter

Preheat oven to 350°. Cook vegetable blend according to package directions; drain. Arrange vegetables in buttered shallow casserole. Combine cream, water, bouillon, and egg in a small saucepan. Stir constantly over medium heat, until hot and slightly thickened; do not overcook. Add mushrooms to cream sauce; pour sauce over vegetables. Top with shredded cheese; sprinkle with salt and pepper. Dot with butter. Bake for 45 minute to 1 hour. Yield: 6 servings.

Cauliflower and Broccoli Casserole
Carbs/serving: 5.39g

2 C. cauliflower florets
2 C. broccoli florets
2 T. butter
1 C. cream
1/4 tsp. salt
1/4 tsp. seasoned salt
1/4 tsp. pepper
1 egg, *beaten*
1 tsp. onion powder
3/4 C. Cheddar cheese, *shredded*
1/2 C. pork rind crumbs, *optional*
Paprika

Preheat oven to 350°. Blanch cauliflower and broccoli separately in boiling, salted water for 1 minute; drain well. Melt butter in small saucepan over medium heat; Stir in cream, salt, seasoned salt, pepper, and egg. Cook, stirring constantly, until thickened. Do not overcook. Add onion powder and cheese, stirring to melt cheese. Layer cauliflower, broccoli and sauce in baking dish; cover with pork rind crumbs, if desired. Sprinkle with paprika. Bake for 30-45 minutes or until vegetables are heated through and sauce is bubbly. Yield: 6 servings.

Stir-Fried Onions and Green Peppers

Carbs/serving: 5.85g

1 1/2 C. onions, *sliced into strips*
2 medium green bell peppers, *seeded and sliced into strips*
1 medium red bell pepper, *seeded and sliced into strips*
3 T. butter or oil

Heat oil or butter in a large skillet over medium-high heat. Sauté onions until golden. Add peppers to onions and continue sautéing until peppers are crisp-tender. Do not over-cook.
Yield: 6 servings.

Fried Cabbage

Carbs/serving: 3.8g

1/4 lb. slab pork, *cut into strips*
4 C. cabbage, *chopped*
Salt and pepper to taste

Fry salt pork in saucepan until crisp; remove from pan. Combine cabbage, salt, pepper, and 1/4 C. water in pork drippings. Simmer, covered, for 10 minutes or until cabbage is tender and begins to brown slightly. Stir occasionally.
Yield: 4 servings.

Sweet and Sour Cabbage

Carbs/serving: 3.35g

4 C. cabbage, *chopped*	1 C. water
2 T. butter	2 T. vinegar
1 tsp. caraway seed	2 pkts. Sweetener
1 tsp. salt	

Combine cabbage, butter, caraway seed, salt, and water in saucepan. Simmer, covered, for 10 minutes or until cabbage is tender. Add vinegar and sweetener; mix lightly.
Yield: 6 servings.

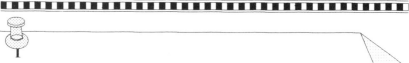

One final note about vegetables: Don't forget about the frozen vegetable blends found in the freezer section of your store. There are several different combinations that are relatively low in carbohydrates and very convenient to make. Simply follow the stove-top or microwave instructions; add some butter and seasonings of your choice, or top with a cheese or alfredo sauce and you have a quick and delicious side-dish to compliment any entree that you prepare. Be sure to check the carb. counts and the ingredient lists. Some "Meal Starter"-type blends include pasta, while others include corn and various beans. Following is a very short list of some blends that we have found. You may find "generic" blends in your local store that will suit you well.

<u>Bird's Eye Brand</u>
Broccoli Stir-Fry 5g/serving
Broccoli, Cauliflower, and Carrots (Californi-style Blend)
                                                               4g/serving
Broccoli, Red Pepper, Onions, Mushrooms 4g/serving
Broccoli, Carrots, and Water Chestnuts 6g/serving
Cauliflower, Carrots, and Snow Peas 6g/serving
Sugar Snap Stir-Fry 6g/serving

<u>Green Giant Brand</u>
California Blend 2g/serving
Heartland Blend 2g/serving
Manhattan Blend 1g/serving
Santa Fe Blend 4g/serving
Seattle Blend 2g/serving

<u>Note</u>: These are only the blends whose carb. counts were 6g/serving or less. There are additional blends whose counts run between 8-15g/serving that might be possibilities for your maintenance plan.

Sauces

Sauces and marinades add a whole new dimension to your meat and vegetable dishes. For the people who tend to use only salt, pepper, and butter for flavoring as they cook, we strongly suggest branching out and experimenting with the following marinades and sauces. Commercial products, as we have said repeatedly throughout this text, are convenient, but tend to contain ingredients that we don't necessarily want to consume. Homemade products, on the other hand, afford you complete control of the ingredients (and therefore, carb. count) but require some additional time in the kitchen. We do ask you, though, to try each of these recipes (especially the barbecue sauces). We think that you will be as excited as we are as to how delicious your foods can taste with minimal carbohydrate impact.

Steak or Chop Marinade

Carbs/Serving: .86g/T.

1/3 C. hot water	1 tsp. beef bouillon granules
2 tsp. onion powder	1 clove garlic, *minced*
2 T. red wine vinegar	1/2 tsp. paprika *(optional)*
2 T. vegetable or olive oil	1/2 tsp. salt
2 T. soy sauce	1/2 tsp. pepper

In a small bowl, combine all ingredients. Set aside until ready to pour over meat for marinating. Yield: Approximately 3/4 cup.
Variation: To use for chicken, substitute chicken bouillon granules for the beef bouillon granules.

Fish Marinade

Carbs/Serving: .12g/T

1/4 C. lemon juice
1/2 C. vegetable or olive oil
1 tsp. salt
1/4 tsp. pepper
1/2 tsp. garlic powder, *optional*

In a small bowl, combine all ingredients. Set aside until ready to pour over fish for marinating. Yield: Approximately 3/4 cup.

Sweet and Smoky Barbecue Sauce

Carbs/Serving: .78g/T

1/2 C. oil
1/2 C. vinegar
1 T. lemon juice
2 T. Worcestershire sauce
1 (8oz.) can tomato sauce
1 T. prepared mustard
Sweetener to equal 1/2 C. sugar
1 tsp. Hot sauce
1 tsp. Liquid Smoke, *optional*

In a medium saucepan, combine all ingredients, mixing well. Cook over low heat, stirring, just until blended and heated through. Allow to cool, and put in jar with screw-top lid, or squeeze bottle. Shake well before each use. Yield: Approximately 2 cups.

Tangy Barbecue Sauce

Carbs/Serving: .90g/T.

1/2 C. oil
1 C. vinegar
1/4 C. water
2 T. paprika
1 tsp. garlic powder
1 tsp. onion salt
1/2 tsp. chili powder
1/4 tsp. cayenne pepper
1 tsp. Hot Sauce
Sweetener to equal 1/2 cup sugar
1 T. cornstarch
1/4 C. cold water

In a medium saucepan, combine first 9 ingredients. Heat over medium heat, stirring frequently. Reduce heat, and add sweetener. Combine cornstarch and cold water. Slowly add cornstarch mixture to sauce, stirring constantly. Continue cooking until sauce is thickened. Allow to cool and put in jar with screw-top lid, or squeeze bottle. Shake well before each use. Yield: Approximately 2 cups.

Meat Pan Gravy

Carbs/Serving: .31g/T.

2 T. meat drippings
2 C. beef or chicken stock (may be made from bouillon granules)
1 T. cornstarch
1/4 C. cold water
Salt, pepper, onion powder to taste

In a saucepan, place meat drippings and stock. Heat over medium heat until bubbly. In a small bowl, combine cornstarch and cold water. Stir into hot stock mixture. Continue cooking and stirring until thickened. Yield: Approximately 2 1/4 cups.

Variations:
Mushroom Gravy Sauce
Carbs/Serving: .56g/T.

1 recipe <u>Meat Pan Gravy</u>
1 T. butter
1 (4oz.) can sliced mushrooms, *drained*
1/2 C. dry red wine, *optional*

In a small pan, melt butter over medium heat. Sauté mushrooms in butter until golden. Stir mushrooms (and wine, if using) into hot meat gravy. Yield: Approximately 2 1/2 cups.

White "Milk" Gravy
Carb/Serving: .56g/T

Following instructions for <u>Meat Pan Gravy</u>, substitute cream for stock. Yield: Approximately 2 1/4 cups.

Cheese Sauce
Carbs/Serving: .62g/T

2 T. butter
1 C. cream
1 T. cornstarch
1/4 C. cold water
1 C. cheddar cheese, *finely shredded*
1/2 tsp. salt
1/8 tsp. paprika, *optional*

In a saucepan, melt butter over medium-low heat. Add cream, and continue heating until hot, but not bubbly. In a small bowl, mix together cornstarch and cold water. Add to hot cream, stirring continually. Add cheese to cream mixture. Continue cooking until cheese is melted and incorporated, and sauce is thickened. Remove from heat and stir in seasonings.
Yield: Approximately 1 3/4 cups.

Variation:

Alfredo Sauce

Carbs/Serving: .63g/T.

Follow the instructions for Cheese Sauce, substituting Parmesan cheese for the cheddar cheese. Add 1/2 tsp. garlic powder, and omit paprika. Yield: Approximately 1 3/4 cups.

> Serve Cheese Sauce over steamed broccoli, cauliflower, asparagus, or (prepared) frozen vegetable blends. For an Italian flare, serve Alfredo Sauce over steamed vegetables as listed above or zucchini squash that has been julienned and lightly sautéed in butter. Wonderful!

Easy Hollandaise Sauce

Carbs/Serving: .11g/T.

3 whole eggs
4 tsp. lemon juice
3 T. water
7 T. butter
1/2 tsp. salt
Pepper to taste, if desired

In a mixing bowl, combine eggs, lemon juice, and water. Whip together until thoroughly blended and pale yellow in color. In a heavy saucepan, melt butter over low heat. Add egg mixture slowly, stirring continuously until sauce has thickened. Do not over cook. Before serving add salt. Season to taste. Yield: Approximately 1 cup. Serve with Eggs Benedict or over steamed broccoli or asparagus spears.

Tartar Sauce

Carbs/Serving: .09g/T.
1 C. mayonnaise
1 tsp. prepared mustard
2 T. dill relish
1-2 pkt. sweetener, optional
1 tsp. horseradish, optional

In a small mixing bowl, combine all ingredients. Mix well. Serve with fried fish or shrimp recipes. Yield: Approximately 1 1/4 cups.

Variation:

Reuben Sauce

Follow instructions for Tartar Sauce except omit: mustard and horseradish. Serve with Reuben Burgers.
Yield: Approximately 1 1/8 cups. (Carbs/Serving: .10g/T.)

Dijon Mayonnaise

Carbs/Serving: .30g/T.
1 C. mayonnaise
2 T. Dijon mustard

In a small bowl, combine together mayonnaise and mustard.
Yield: 1 1/8 cups.

Herb-Flavored Mayonnaise

Carbs/Serving: .10g/T.
1 C. mayonnaise
1/2 tsp. garlic powder
1 tsp. Worcestershire sauce
1/2 tsp. basil
1/2 tsp. dill
1/2 tsp. tarragon

In a small bowl, combine together all ingredients.
Yield: Approximately 1 1/8 cups.

Commercial Sauces and Seasonings

This is certainly not an exhaustive list of the many types or brands of sauces and seasonings available on the market today. However, it may give you a start, and help steer you into the sauces, seasonings, and marinades sections of your favorite store. Caution: These products are quick and convenient, and we've picked the "lesser of the evils" in terms of carb. counts. But, for the most part they all contain some amount of sugar. So, be careful and use them only as they fit into your eating plan!

Brown Gravy/Pork Gravy Sauces or Mixes
Franco-American 4g/serving
Heinz 3g/serving
Durkee or French's (Mix) 3g/serving
Knorr Classic (Mix) 3g/serving
McCormick (Mix) 3g/serving

Mushroom Gravy Sauces
Franco-American (Brown) 3g/serving
(Creamy) 4g/serving
Pepperidge Farm (Country Mushroom or with wine) 4g/serving

Chicken/Turkey Gravy Sauces or Mixes
Franco-American (Original) 3/serving
(Giblet) 3g/serving
Heinz (Homestyle Classic) 3g/serving
Pepperidge Farm (Cream of) 3g/serving
(Golden) 3g/serving
(Rotisserie) 3g/serving
Durkee, French's, McCormick (Mix) 4g/serving
Weight Watcher's (Mix) 1g/serving

Stroganoff Gravy and Mix
Pepperidge Farm 4g/serving

Alfredo Sauces
Five Brother's Alfredo and Creamy Pesto Sauce 2g/serving
Five Brother's Alfredo w/Mushroom 3g/serving
Ragu's Alfredo Sauce 3g/serving

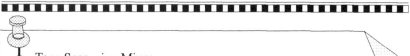

Taco Seasoning Mixes
Ortega 4g/serving
Durkee 2g/serving
Fajita Seasoning Mixes
Ortega 3g/serving
Lawry's 3g/serving
Taco Sauces
Ortega and Old El Paso 1 g/1 T.
Chi Chi's Thick and Chunky 1g/1 T.
Steak Sauces
A.1. Steak Sauce 2g/1 T.
Hunt's Steak Sauce 2g/1 T.
Old Smokehouse Steak Sauce
London Pub Steak and Chop Sauce 2.8g/1 T.

Barbecue Sauces
Hunt's Light 6g/2 T.
Healthy Choice (all varieties) 6g/2 T.
Heinz Buffalo Wings 4g/2 T.
Porino's Italian 7g/2 T.
House of Tsang Hong Kong 2g/1 tsp.
Barbecue Seasoning
Durkee 0g/1/4 tsp.
Meat and Vegetable Seasonings
Prudhomme's   Blackened Steak 0g/serving
                Vegetable Magic 0g/serving
                Meat Magic   0g/serving
Mesquite Sauce
S & W 3g/1T.
Mesquite Seasoning
Tone's (Butter) 0g/1/4 tsp.
Mexican Seasoning
Tone's 1.3g/1 tsp.
Chi-Chi's Mix 1g/1 tsp.
Dry Seasoning Mixes by Sun-Bird
Stir-Fry 3g/serving
Lemon Chicken Stir-fry 3g/serving
Chow Mein 3g/serving

Desserts

Desserts, in our humble opinion, are a needed component of any phase of a low-carbohydrate eating plan. Please let us explain! Sometimes we would crave something on the sweet side, and having a "legal", lower-carbohydrate dessert at the ready would keep us out of the cookie jar. Other times, simply knowing that we were not deprived of desserts was enough to satisfy us psychologically—you know, the "forbidden fruit" syndrome.

During the weight-loss phase of our eating programs, however, we did limit ourselves to the number of desserts served per week. And then, we arranged our meal plans for the day to account for the additional carbs. that we would have with the dessert (and extra cup of coffee).

Also, we found it very useful to have a variety of dessert recipes so that if we were invited to someone's home for dinner or a church potluck, we could say "I'll bring a dessert", and know that we were taking something that would not throw us off the path. Our friends have made the comment, "Oh, this dessert is so good! I'm sorry that you messed up your diet tonight by eating this." To which we would just smile and reply, "But, this *is* a "diet" dessert. It has no sugar added." We think that you'll enjoy the incredulous stares of your friends and family as much as we do.

Gelatin desserts are so versatile! With the many flavors available in sugar-free form, you can vary and change a dessert a myriad of ways. With any gelatin dessert, be sure to allow yourself plenty of time (perhaps up to 2 days in advance of serving) to prepare the dish.

Layered Gelatin Dessert

Carbs/Serving: 3.70g

2 lg. (8-1/2 cup serving size) pkg. sugar-free gelatin dessert mix, *any flavor*
4 C. hot water, *divided*
1 pkg. plain Knox gelatin
1/4 C. cold water
Sweetener to equal 1 C. sugar
1 C. whipping cream
1(16 oz.) carton sour cream

In a small mixing bowl, stir together until thoroughly mixed: 1 pkg. gelatin mix and 2 C. hot water. Pour into a 9x13" pan and place in refrigerator until set, 2-3 hours. When set, prepare second layer:

Dissolve plain gelatin in 1/4 C. cold water; set aside. In a small saucepan, mix together sweetener and whipping cream. Heat the cream mixture to a light simmer, but do not boil. Take off heat, cool to room temperature. Stir in gelatin mixture and sour cream. Pour over first set gelatin layer. Return to refrigerator to allow to set, another 2-3 hours.

When set, prepare third layer as you did the first with the remaining package of gelatin and 2 C. hot water. Allow to cool to room temperature. Pour over first two layers. Return to refrigerator to set, another 2-3 hours. Yield: 12 servings.

Note: For a more festive, "circus-striped" appearance, you might make each gelatin layer of different flavors. (What about lime and strawberry layers for Christmas?) Have fun!

Gelatin Parfaits

Carbs/Serving: 3.02g

2 sm. (4-1/2 cup serving size) pkg. sugar-free gelatin dessert mix, *any flavor or combination of two flavors*
1 C. cream, *with sweetener added to equal 1/4 cup sugar and whipped to firm peaks*

Prepare gelatin according to package directions. (You may prepare two flavors separately for a multi-color parfait.) When gelatin is set, spoon out 1/2 the gelatin (or 1 flavor gelatin) into 4 dessert glasses. Spoon into the glasses a layer of whipped cream. Top the cream with the remaining gelatin (or second flavor gelatin). Garnish parfait with a dollop of the whipped cream. Yield: 4 servings

Whipped Cream Fluff

Carbs/Serving: 1.65g

2 C. whipping cream
1 sm. (4 1/2 C. serving-size) pkg. gelatin dessert mix, *any flavor*

In a large mixing bowl, pour in cream. With an electric mixer, whip cream until it begins to thicken. As you continue to whip the cream, sprinkle dry gelatin mixture over cream to mix it in. Continue whipping until soft peaks form. (Do not overbeat, or the results will be a dry mixture resembling cottage cheese curds.) Yield: 8 servings.

Variation: Before whipping cream, place 1 (8oz.) pkg. cream cheese into mixing bowl. Beat cheese until smooth. Add cream slowly to cream cheese, mixing to thoroughly blend. Continue recipe instructions as above. Yield: 8 servings. (Carbs/Serving: 2.56g)

Sweetened Cream Cheese Balls

Carbs/Serving: 3.54g

1 (8oz.) pkg. cream cheese, *softened*
Sweetener to equal 1/4 C. sugar
Sweetened Cinnamon (Recipe follows)

Mix cream cheese and sweetener thoroughly. (If the cream cheese mixture is too soft to handle, place in the refrigerator for 10-15 minutes to re-chill.) Pinch off small amounts of the cream cheese mixture and roll in the palms of your hands to form balls about the size of a large marble. In a small bowl, put 2 tablespoons of Sweetened Cinnamon. Roll each cream cheese ball in the cinnamon until coated. Yield: 8 servings (Approximately 2 balls/serving).

Sweetened Cinnamon

Carbs/Serving: 1.3 g/1/2 tsp.

2 T. cinnamon
Sweetener to equal 1/2 C. sugar

Mix cinnamon and sweetener together and store in an air-tight container. Use this as a coating for the cream cheese balls (above) or sprinkle lightly over egg custard, ice cream, or cheesecake as a wonderful topping. (Yield: Approximately 18 1/2 tsp. servings.

Note: Once you are on the Maintenance level of your eating program, and you allow yourself some low-carb. bread products, you can sprinkle Sweetened Cinnamon over buttered toast for a low-carb. version of Cinnamon toast!

Variations of Sweetened Cream Cheese Balls:

Cinnamon-Nut Balls

Add 1/4 C. ground nut topping to the sweetened cinnamon before coating the cream cheese balls. This will raise the carb/serving count to 4.29g (provided that you use the entire coating mixture—which you probably will not).

Peanut Butter Balls

Carbs/Serving: 4.13g

Following the instructions and ingredients for Sweetened Cream Cheese Balls, add 2 tablespoons smooth peanut butter*, and 1 T. baking cocoa. Increase the sweetener to be equal to 1/2 cup sugar. Omit the Sweetened Cinnamon and roll the balls in a chopped nut topping. Yield: 9 servings (Approximately 2 balls/serving)

*Some peanut butters can be an unnecessarily sugared concoction. Some of the better choices available, in terms of carb. count, are as follows:

Adams Natural or No-Stir Peanut Butter 4g/2 T.
Peter Pan Real or Whipped Peanut Butter 5g/2 T.
Roaster Fresh or Unsalted 5g/2 T.

Once again, let us state: Be sure to avoid peanut butters tagged as low- or reduced-fat. You're sure to double the carbohydrate count!

Peanut Butter Pie

Carbs/Serving: 6.01g

1 pkg. plain Knox gelatin
1/2 C. cold water
1/2 C. cream
1 (8oz.) pkg. cream cheese, *softened*
1/2 C. peanut butter
Sweetener to equal 1/2 C. sugar
1 C. cream, *whipped to soft peaks*

Dissolve plain gelatin in 1/2 C. cold water; set aside. In a small saucepan, pour in 1/2 C. cream. Heat cream to a light simmer, but do not boil. Add gelatin to heated cream. Pour cream mixture into a large mixing bowl. Using an electric mixer, mix together cream mixture, cream cheese, peanut butter, and sweetener. Place in refrigerator until mixture just begins to thicken. (See Caution 1, pg. 158.) When it is *slightly* thickened, fold into the mixture the whipped cream. Spoon this into a 9" pie plate. Return to the refrigerator until set, about 3-4 hours. Yield: 8 servings.

Cheesecake

Carbs/Serving: 4.84g

2 (8oz.) pkg. cream cheese, *softened*
Sweetener to equal 3/4 C. sugar
3 eggs
2 tsp. vanilla

Preheat oven to 300°. Cream cheese and sweetener thoroughly. Add eggs, one at a time, beating well after each addition. Stir in vanilla. Pour into a buttered 9" pie pan. Place pie pan into a large baking pan; pour hot water around the pie pan to a depth of 1". Bake for 45 minutes or until firm. Remove from oven and hot water bath. Allow to cool on counter for 20 minutes, then place in refrigerator overnight. Serve chilled. Yield: 8 servings.

Vanilla Ice Cream

Carbs/Serving: 5.91g

4 C. cream, *divided*
Sweetener to equal 3/4 C. sugar
1/8 tsp. salt
1 1/2 tsp. vanilla

In a small saucepan, scald (but do not boil), 1 cup cream. Stir in sweetener, salt, and vanilla until well blended. Remove from heat, pour into the freezer canister of your ice-cream freezer or churn, and place in the refrigerator to chill. When chilled, add remaining 3 cups of cream. Churn the ice cream according to the manufacturer's directions of your ice cream freezer.
Yield: 8 servings.

Variation:

Ice Cream Float

1 recipe Vanilla Ice Cream
Flavored Diet Soda

Scoop ice cream into a tall glass, and pour soda over all. Serve with a spoon and a straw. Yield: 8 servings (Carb count doesn't change).

You may choose to invest in a small electric ice-cream freezer (Oster™ is one possible brand) that uses table salt and refrigerator ice-cubes. It sits on your counter and can make 1 recipe of ice cream in approximately 15-20 minutes. Making and serving ice cream on a moment's notice, any time of the year is no trouble at all. Your children and your sweet tooth will love you for it!

Chocolate Bombe

Carbs/Serving: 5.06g

1 1/2 tsp. Knox unflavored gelatin
1 C. cold water
3 C. cream, *divided*
Sweetener to equal 1 C. sugar
2 T. cocoa
1 tsp. vanilla

Combine gelatin and cold water; set aside. In a small saucepan, scald 1 C. cream; stir in sweetener and cocoa. Add to this mixture the gelatin. Remove from heat and allow to cool. Add vanilla. Pour into a medium mixing bowl and allow to chill until just cool to the touch. Whip remaining 2 cups cream until thickened but not stiff. Fold whipped cream into thickened gelatin mixture. Line a mold or rounded bowl with plastic wrap (to ease removal of the bombe at serving time). Spoon cream mixture into the lined, chilled mold or rounded bowl, packing firmly so that there are no air pockets. Cover mold or bowl and place in freezer at least 6 hours, but no longer than 24-48 hours. Remove from freezer 1/2 hour before serving. Leave in mold until time to serve. Then, turn the bombe out onto a chilled serving plate by running the mold briefly under cool water to help loosen it. Yield: 10 servings.

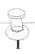

Caution 1: When creating recipes with gelatin such as Chocolate Bombe or Bavarian Cream Puddings, be careful to allow heated mixtures to cool in the refrigerator just long enough so that they will not melt the whipped cream to be incorporated. If allowed to cool too long, you will wind up with a stiff jiggler^{TM}-like product!

Bavarian Cream Pudding

Carbs/Serving: 4.52g

1 pkt. Knox unflavored gelatin	2 tsp. vanilla
1/2 C. cold water	2 C. heavy whipping cream,
5 eggs, *slightly beaten*	*whipped to soft peaks*
Sweetener to equal 1/2 C. sugar	

Dissolve gelatin in cold water; set aside. In the top of a double-boiler, over—not in—*gently* boiling water, place eggs and sweetener. Beat eggs and sweetener as they heat for 7 minutes, or until egg mixture begins to thicken. Remove from heat. Add gelatin mixture. Place in a medium mixing bowl, and place in refrigerator until just cooled. When cool, stir in vanilla. Fold in whipped cream. Chill the mixture until it is like heavy cream. Yield: 6 servings.

Variations:

Lemon Bavarian Pudding

Following the instructions for Bavarian Cream Pudding, add to heated eggs and sweetener mixture, 1-2 T. lemon juice. (Carbs and servings remain the same.)

Chocolate Bavarian Pudding

Carbs/Serving: 5.52g

Following the instructions for Bavarian Cream Pudding, add to heated eggs and sweetener mixture, 2 T. baking cocoa. Yield: 6 servings.

Caution 2: When cooking egg mixtures over a double-boiler, be certain that water is simmering or gently boiling, and that they are cooked just until hot through and beginning to thicken. If the eggs are cooked over too-high heat or for too long, you'll just wind up with scrambled eggs!

Egg custard

Carbs/Serving: 4.32g

2 C. cream
Sweetener to equal 1/2 cup sugar
1/8 tsp. salt
3 eggs, *slightly beaten*
1/2 tsp. vanilla

Preheat oven to 300°. Combine together all ingredients, and pour into a 9" pie plate or into individual custard cups. Place the pie plate or cups into a large pan and pour hot water around these to a depth of 1". Bake custard for 1 hour (or more) if using pie plate; 20-30 minutes for cups or until done. Custard will be done when a knife inserted halfway between center and edge comes out clean. Remove from oven and hot water bath. Allow to cool before serving. Yield: 6 servings.

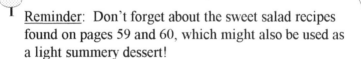

Reminder: Don't forget about the sweet salad recipes found on pages 59 and 60, which might also be used as a light summery dessert!

Some Final Thoughts from the Authors

From Theresa:
I am a 31 year old mother of 2, who had tried every "diet" plan known to man. Until now, my success rate had been almost nil. Now, I don't "diet". I made a "lifestyle change" which has resulted in placing me on the steady track of a thinner, healthier me (at the time of this first printing, I have lost 25 pounds in the course of just two short months). When I started watching my carbohydrate count instead of fat grams, I not only started losing inches, but everyone kept asking me, "What have you done? Your cheeks are so rosy, and your hair is so thick and shiny." This lifestyle has turned my life around. When I went to the doctor to get blood work done, my cholesterol levels and HDL levels were "wonderful". The doctor couldn't believe it! Tracy and I both realize that all of the "low carb" diet plans available on the market today are still a bit controversial, but for the two of us it has been a fantastic lifestyle change. That's why we wanted to share our change with you. We compiled these recipes so you and your family could see how easy it is to change your lifestyle without having to give up many of your favorite foods. I want to personally thank you for purchasing our book and wish you all the best in using it. I hope that your lifestyle change is as easy as mine has been.

From Tracy:
I am a 35 year old mother of 3 who, like Theresa, had no lasting success on any "popular" diet plan on the market today. When I was introduced to the concept of low-carbohydrate dieting, I was skeptical. Now, having lost 30 pounds and 6 dress sizes in approximately 7 months with no struggle or hunger, I am a firm believer. I echo all of the sentiments of Theresa. I look and feel healthier than I ever have before. Thank you for allowing us to share our experiences and recipes with you. We wish you the best and greatest success with your low-carbohydrate lifestyle. Get the mind-set and stay "low-carbing"! In the immortal words of Winston Churchill, "Never give up! Never give up! Never, never, never give up!"

Index

Appetizers and Snacks
Appetizer Pie, 32
Barbecue-Sauced Meatballs, 26
Barbecued Chicken-Little "Legs", 36
Basic Stuffed Mushrooms, 27
Beefy Cheese Ball, 32
Buffalo Chicken Wings, 36
Buttermilk-Ranch Chicken Spread, 33
Cheesy Bacon Cheese Ball, 32
Chili con Queso, 28
Fried Cheese Sticks, 35
Fun Gelatin Squares, 37
Guacamole, 29
Ham and Cheese Ball, 31
Ham Roll-Ups, 33
Ham-Stuffed Mushrooms, 27
Make-a-Dip-in-a-Flash, 30
Marinated Cheese and Olives, 34
Marinated Mozzarella, 34
Oven-Roasted Chili Brie, 35
Party Cheese Ball, 31
Pepperoni-Stuffed Mushrooms, 27
Salami Roll-Ups, 34
Salsa Dip, 28
Sausage-Stuffed Mushrooms, 27
Seafood-Stuffed Mushrooms 27
Spicy Cheese Dip for Vegetables, 29
Sweetened Stuffing for Celery Sticks, 37

Beverages. Information about,
Beverage Mixes, 40
Diet Soda, 41
Flavored Coffees, 41
Flavored Teas, 40
Flavored Waters, 39, 40

Salads and Dressings
Bean Sprout Salad, 51
Caesar Chicken Salad, 56
Carrot-Pineapple Gelatin Salad, 59
Cauliflower-Lettuce-Bacon Salad, 53
Cauliflower "Potato" Salad, 53
Chinese Chicken Salad, 57
Chinese Coleslaw, 49

Salads and Dressings, continued:
Cole Slaw, 47
Creamy Coleslaw, 49
Creamy Cucumber Dressing, 61
Creamy Italian Dressing, 62
Crunchy Chicken Salad, 57
Deb's Cucumbers, 50
French Dressing, 61
Fried Chicken Salad, 55
Ham and Cheese Salad, 58
Hearty Italian Salad, 46
Hot Chicken Salad, 56
Hot Green Bean Salad, 51
Layered Lettuce Salad, 46
1-Minute Caesar Salad, 45
Orange or Lime Fluff, 60
Parmesan Dressing, 61
St. Louis Salad, 52
Salad of a Million Faces, The, 44
Strawberry and Rhubarb Salad Molds, 59
Summer Salad, 52
Taco Salad, 54
Theresa's Vinegar-Mustard Dressing, 62
Tuna Salad, 58
Vinaigrette Dressing, 62
Vinegar Cucumber Salad, 50
Wilted Salad, 47

Meaty Main Dishes

Poultry, 65
Bacon-Cheddar Chicken Rolls, 73
Baked Chicken, 66
Broiled Lemon Pepper Chicken Wings, 65
Cheddar-Sauced Chicken Breasts, 68
Chicken Amandine, 77
Chicken Breasts Stuffed with Mozzarella, 71
Chicken Chow Mein, 79
Chicken Cordon Bleu, 67
Chicken Dijon, 82
Chicken "Enchiladas", 70
Chicken in Cream Sauce, 78
Chicken Kiev, 73
Chicken Monterey, 77

Meaty Main Dishes, Continued
Poultry, Continued
Chicken Nuggets, 75
Chicken Paprika, 84
Chicken Rolls Amandine, 74
Chicken with Lemon Sauce, 83
Crunchy Fried Chicken Breasts, 76
Garlic Chicken, 80
Grilled Marinated Chicken Breasts, 76
Herb-Marinated Chicken, 81
Italian-Style Chicken Breasts, 70
Mushroom and Swiss Chicken Breasts, 70
Pan-Fried Chicken Breasts, 68
Roast Turkey Breast, 84
Royal Barbecued Chicken, 82
Santa Fe Chicken, 81
Sesame Chicken, 78
Tarragon-Sauced Chicken Breasts, 69
Turkey Stir-Fry, 84
Beef, 85
Barbecued Beef Pot Roast, 93
Beef Goulash, 100
Border Chili, 89
Cheeseburgers, 86
Country-Fried Steak, 97
Fajitas, 98
Gravy-Sauced Meatballs, 90
Hamburgers, 85
Herbed Rump Roast, 94
Italian Beef, 95
Marinated steaks, 96
Meatloaf, 88
Mushroom Swiss Burgers, 87
Pizza burgers, 86
Pot Roast, 92
Ranch burgers, 86
Reuben Burgers, 91
Salisbury Steak, 87
Sloppy Joes, 90
Southwest Casserole, 89
Steak and Green Peppers, 99
Steak Roll with Dressing, 101
Stroganoff, 88
Swedish Meatballs, 91
Swiss Steak, 99
Taco burgers, 87
Pork, 102
Baked Ham, 109
Baked Pork Chops, 104
Barbecued Pork Roast, 103
Barbecued Pork Steak, 107
Breaded Fried Pork Chops, 105
Breaded Pork Cutlets (with Pan Gravy), 106
Broiled or Grilled Pork Chops, 105

Pork, Continued
Country-Style Ribs, 108
Grilled Italian Sausages, 110
Ham Steak, 110
Italian Sausage "Burgers", 112
Mediterranean Pork, 109
Polish Sausage and Sauerkraut, 112
Pork Chow Mein, 108
Pork Roast, 102
Pork Roast Stir-Fry, 104
Sautéed Pork Chops, 104
Side Pork, 112
Stuffed Bratwurst, 111
Fish, 113
Baked Fish with Mushrooms, 113
"Blackened" Fish Fillets, 113
Cajun Catfish Fillets, 114
Fish Fillets Amandine, 116
Fried Popcorn Shrimp, 117
Shrimp in Garlic Butter, 117
Southwestern Grilled Fish, 115
Tuna Patties, 116

Eggs
Cheese and Onion Scrambled Eggs, 121
Chiles Rellenos Casserole, 125
Crustless Quiche, 124
Devilled Eggs, 119
Dinner Omelets, 122
Eggs Benedict, 126
Eggs in Bacon Rings, 127
Eggs in Ham Cakes, 127
Egg-Sausage Stir-Fry, 126
Filling Suggestions for Omelets, 123
  —Cheese filling, 123
  —Denver filling, 123
  —Mushroom filling, 123
Italian Herbed Scrambled Eggs, 122
Mushroom Scrambled Eggs, 121
Quiche Lorraine, 124
Western (or Denver) Scrambled Eggs, 121

Vegetables
Asparagus Amandine, 135
Asparagus in Cheese Sauce, 136
"Batter"-Fried Vegetables, 134
Broccoli-Carrot Stir-Fry, 137
California Casserole, 140
Cauliflower and Broccoli Casserole, 140
Cauliflower in Cheese Sauce, 138
Cauliflower with Almond Butter, 139
Chinese Broccoli, 138
Classic Green Beans, 130

Vegetables, Continued
Fried Cabbage, 141
Fried Cauliflower with Cheese Sauce, 139
Green Beans in Herbed Butter, 130
Green Beans Amandine, 131
Golden Broccoli Bake, 137
Herb-Buttered Mushrooms, 132
Sautéed Mushrooms, 132
Sesame Asparagus, 135
Spanish-Style Green Beans, 131
Stir-Fried Onions and Green Peppers, 141
Stir-Fried Squash, 133
Sweet and Sour Cabbage, 141
Winning Vegetables, 136
Zucchini in Dill Sauce, 133
Zucchini Patties, 134

Sauces
Alfredo Sauce, 147
Cheese Sauce, 146
Dijon Mayonnaise, 148
Easy Hollandaise Sauce, 147
Fish Marinade, 144
Herb-Flavored Mayonnaise, 148
Meat Pan Gravy, 145
Mushroom Gravy Sauce, 146
Reuben Sauce, 148
Steak or Chop Marinade, 143
Sweet and Smoky Barbecue Sauce, 144
Tangy Barbecue Sauce, 145
Tartar Sauce, 148
White "Milk" Gravy, 146

Desserts
Bavarian Cream Pudding, 159
Cheesecake, 156
Chocolate Bavarian Pudding, 159
Chocolate Bombe, 158
Cinnamon-Nut Balls, 155
Egg Custard, 160
Gelatin Parfaits, 153
Ice Cream Floats, 157
Layered Gelatin Dessert, 152
Lemon Bavarian Pudding, 159
Peanut Butter Balls, 155
Peanut Butter Pie, 156
Sweetened Cinnamon, 154
Sweetened Cream Cheese Balls, 154
Whipped Cream Fluff, 153
Vanilla Ice Cream, 157

Thank you for purchasing Easy Living Low-Carb Cooking.
If you wish to order more copies, please visit **www.carbsmart.com**
or fill in the form below. Please make checks payable to CarbSmart, Inc.
Payment Method: ❏ Cash   ❏ Check   ❏ Credit Card

_____ copies of *Easy Living Low-Carb Cooking* $14.99 each   _____
         Plus Shipping and Handling   First book add $3.95   _____
                         then $1.00 each additional copy $ _____

                                     Total Enclosed $ _____
Mail To: CarbSmart, Inc. • 1335 Greg Street, Suite 106 • Sparks, NV 89431
❏ Visa   ❏ MasterCard   ❏ American Express   ❏ Discover

Card Number _____ Exp. Date ___/___

Name _____

Address _____

City_____ State_____ Zip_____

Phone: _____ E-mail: _____

- -

Thank you for purchasing Easy Living Low-Carb Cooking.
If you wish to order more copies, please visit **www.carbsmart.com**
or fill in the form below. Please make checks payable to CarbSmart, Inc.
Payment Method: ❏ Cash   ❏ Check   ❏ Credit Card

_____ copies of *Easy Living Low-Carb Cooking* $14.99 each   _____
         Plus Shipping and Handling   First book add $3.95   _____
                         then $1.00 each additional copy $ _____

                                     Total Enclosed $ _____
Mail To: CarbSmart, Inc. • 1335 Greg Street, Suite 106 • Sparks, NV 89431
❏ Visa   ❏ MasterCard   ❏ American Express   ❏ Discover

Card Number _____ Exp. Date ___/___

Name _____

Address _____

City_____ State_____ Zip_____

Phone: _____ E-mail: _____